Paula Newby-Fraser's
Peak Fitness
for Women

Paula Newby-Fraser
with
John M. Mora

Human Kinetics

Library of Congress Cataloging-in-Publication Data

Newby-Fraser, Paula, 1962-
 [Peak fitness for women]
 Paula Newby-Fraser's peak fitness for women / Paula Newby-Fraser
with John Mora.
  p.   cm.
 Includes bibliographical references and index.
 ISBN 0-87322-672-0 (pbk.)
 1. Physical fitness for women. I. Mora, John, 1964- .
II. Title. III. Title: Peak fitness for women.
 GV482.N48   1995
 613.7'045--dc20   94-40070
                                                            CIP

ISBN: 0-87322-672-0

Developmental Editors: Mary E. Fowler and Dawn Roselund; **Assistant Editors:** Kirby Mittelmeier, Henry Woolsey, and Erik Dafforn; **Copyeditor:** Barbara Field; **Proofreader:** Pam Johnson; **Indexer:** Margie Towery; **Typesetting & Layout Artists:** Kathleen Boudreau-Fuoss and Denise Lowry; **Text Designer:** Stuart Cartwright; **Cover Designer:** Jack Davis; **Cover Photographer:** John Mora; **Illustrator:** Tara Welsch; **Printer:** Versa Press

Human Kinetics books are available at special discounts for bulk purchase. Special editions or book excerpts can also be created to specification. For details, contact the Special Sales Manager at Human Kinetics.

Printed in the United States of America   10   9   8   7   6   5   4   3

Human Kinetics
Web site: http: // www.humankinetics.com/

United States: Human Kinetics, P.O. Box 5076, Champaign, IL 61825-5076
1-800-747-4457

Canada: Human Kinetics, Box 24040, Windsor, ON N8Y 4Y9
1-800-465-7301 (in Canada only)

Europe: Human Kinetics, P.O. Box IW14, Leeds LS16 6TR, United Kingdom
(44) 1132 781708

Australia: Human Kinetics, 57A Price Avenue, Lower Mitcham, South Australia 5062
(08) 277 1555

New Zealand: Human Kinetics, P.O. Box 105-231, Auckland 1
(09) 523 3462

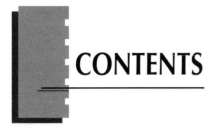

CONTENTS

FOREWORD

Lives of several women have inspired me to new levels within my own. The timeless pastels of Georgia O'Keefe, painted from her home in northern New Mexico, have opened creative doors within me that for years had been hidden. Dian Fossey's commitment to the mountain gorillas, a cause that eventually cost her her life, continually fuels me to stay tuned to my own purpose, my own heart. Not all of my heroines are people who exist beyond the bounds of my own life, however. There is one who has crossed my path many times over. And that heroine is Paula Newby-Fraser.

Paula and I have been both comrades *and* competitors for nearly a decade. Many classic duels between us out on the race course have passed under the bridge. Some of them were friendly challenges; most, however, were all-guts-no-glitter affairs. It was during those battles that I saw in Paula the commitment of a Dian Fossey that makes her a winner. I saw the creativity of a Georgia O'Keefe that allowed Paula to hone her body into art-in-motion. But I also saw something else in Paula—a commitment to a lifestyle that doesn't end once she crosses the finish line.

Paula's career has been sculpted by hard work, passion, and an unwillingness to accept other people's ideas of what is possible. She has used athletics as a way to explore and express herself. She has always approached sport with passion, not obsession. She doesn't brag about her accomplishments.

I invite you to enjoy her book *Paula Newby-Fraser's Peak Fitness for Women.* She will take you through everything: the nuts and bolts of getting started, the developing of a sensible training program, the many considerations of how to schedule your workouts into the demands of the real world, and perfecting your athletic performance. You will find plenty of inspiration, a lot of great information, and enough motivation to set you on your way to a lifestyle where health and happiness are one and the same.

Julie Moss
Editor, *Competitor for Women Magazine*
and former world-class triathlete

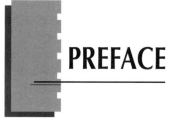

PREFACE

Do you want to go beyond—perhaps far beyond—your current fitness level? Have you ever experienced glimpses, however fleeting, of your true athletic potential, and wondered what it would take to realize that potential?

"Peak fitness" is all about reaching your potential. And *Paula Newby-Fraser's Peak Fitness for Women* gives you what you need to do just that.

If you're a "serious" female athlete, whatever your current fitness level, you know that knowledge is the key to greater performance. In this book, I'll give you advanced techniques and sophisticated training secrets that have helped me go from a beginning runner to a seven-time Ironman Triathlon champion.

But peak fitness isn't just for triathletes. Whether you run, cycle, lift weights, in-line skate, or perform aerobics, the information provided here will help you soar beyond your current fitness limitations. Throughout this book, I will share proven training methods designed and taught by some of the foremost experts and coaches in the area of sports physiology.

This book takes a progressive approach. Chapters 1 and 2 set the foundation for peak fitness. You'll learn about many of the benefits of high-level fitness, some of which you may find surprising. You'll learn the secret of the Peak Fitness Triangle, which will define the essential training components that will help you reach your fitness goals. Finally, you'll discover the necessary investments—emotional, financial, and otherwise—needed for the exciting journey ahead.

Chapters 3 through 5 provide the practical, no-nonsense training knowledge you need. These chapters provide examples, illustrations, and numerous photos that will help guide you to your target.

The remainder of the book helps you put it all together in a useful, manageable way. You'll learn about the importance of the mental side of training, the value of resting for better subsequent performances, and what you need to know about your unique nutrition needs. In addition, you'll discover the key workout method, an innovative, time-efficient way to schedule your workouts within your busy lifestyle. Finally, you'll learn how to endure all that hard training and still be sharp, fresh, and primed for peak performance at your next race or competition.

You'll also find this book a functional workbook that will help you measure and track your progress. Blank log pages and sample training templates are included within the book, and the information in the appendix will help guide you to more valuable resources.

And because everyone needs a little motivation along the way, I've provided some valuable personal insight throughout the book, taken from over a decade of training and professional racing. I'll tell you about some of the mistakes I've made and (I hope) help you to avoid them.

I congratulate you for taking the first step toward what may be unknown territory for you. No matter what your fitness goal, *Paula Newby-Fraser's Peak Fitness for Women* will guide you through the exciting frontier of female athletic performance. More importantly, it will help you reach your full athletic potential.

Paula Newby-Fraser

To my parents. For the tremendous diversity they provided me that somehow bred balance.

P.N.F.

To every wonderful person who has sweated and toiled in a swimming pool, on a bicycle seat, or on a running trail in celebration of life.

J.M.M.

ACKNOWLEDGMENTS

Much of my success as a professional triathlete has been due to the various opportunities I've had to draw on experts in specialized fields related to peak fitness. I'd like to acknowledge the following people for contributing their technical expertise to this book: Diane Buchta, Dr. Donna Brown, Julian Littleford, Dr. Glenn Town, Dr. Darryl Hobson, Dr. John Ivy, Dr. Michael Sherman, Rob Sleamaker, Monique Ryan, Dr. J. Kenney, Dr. Jeffrey Blumberg, Dr. Kathleen Zechmeister, Dr. J.P. Neary, Dr. Owen Anderson, and Dr. Morris Mann. I'd especially like to thank Diane Buchta for the use of her comprehensive weight training program and for all her help in putting that chapter together.

Thanks to the folks at *Peak Performance Running* newsletter, *The Total Triathlon Almanac*, and *Running Research News* for letting us use and adapt some chart materials.

Thanks also to the staff at the Bedford Park Library in Bedford Park, Illinois for its help in doing research and obtaining copies of books, articles, and journal studies. Special thanks to professional researcher Margaret Stepien for her support, encouragement, and fax machine.

From the video production people who allowed us to use the log page layouts, I'd like to thank Kevin Wendle, John Bult, and Newt Walker.

Many of my triathlon colleagues contributed their experience and added valuable insight to many topics in the book: Mark Allen, Karen Smyers, Joanne Ritchey, Sixto Linares, Wolfgang Dittrich, Jurgen Zack, Paul Huddle, and Todd Jacobs.

Our gratitude to the many others who contributed in various aspects of putting the book together: Tony Svensson for his help in putting together training schedules; Shelley Berryhill from *Windy City Sports* for her outstanding proofreading and editing skills; Paul Barton from The Camera Stop for his great studio shots in the stretching chapter; Aislinn Wiley, Lauren Jensen, Kara Hughes, and Liz LaPlante for modeling; Janet Wendle for modeling in the strength training chapter; and Ted Miller at Human Kinetics for helping to conceive and produce this book and his contagious enthusiasm through its early stages.

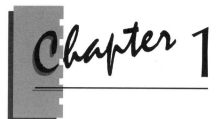

Achieving Peak Fitness as a Woman

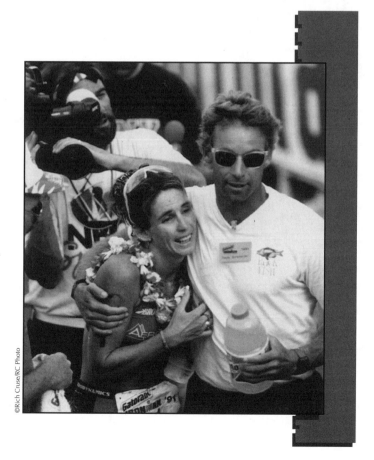

©Rich Cruse/RC Photo

To encourage those of you who aren't sure just how serious you are, or who doubt that you can achieve peak fitness, I'll tell you about my average beginnings in professional endurance sports.

THE ROAD TO HAWAII

In 1983, in my hometown of Durban, South Africa, I was a different woman with a vastly different lifestyle. After graduating from college, I began working a 9-to-5 job as a researcher in a property management firm.

I worked in a competitive, all-female department where job performance was often measured by who wore the most stylish clothes or who caught the most approving stares from the male employees in other departments. I spent lunch hours in boutiques and clothing stores shopping for the latest eye-catching fashions with my co-worker and close friend, Adele.

My weekends were as predictable as the sunset. Every Friday night, a group of us swayed our hips at a popular dance club until early Saturday morning. The rest of the weekend we sunbathed on the beach, fulfilling our quest for the ultimate tan. An occasional stroll through knee-deep water was our only exercise.

During one of our lunch-hour shopping sprees, Adele suggested that we start jogging. Although the idea seemed preposterous, it came at a point when I was gaining weight, so, plagued by the rubber tire inflating around my hips, I gave her the nod.

We jogged three times a week before work, sweating off those extra pounds that threatened to forestall our live-for-the-weekend lifestyle. Adele would wait for me up the road from my house at 6:00 a.m. every morning, providing the incentive I needed; I didn't want to leave her standing on the street in the dark.

Within a few weeks, I found myself looking forward to jogging, and gradually my motivation to run changed. Where at first I had run in the hope of fitting into a smaller swimsuit size, I now ran for sheer pleasure, for the exhilaration I felt when pushing hard. My sessions became longer and faster, and I started to run afternoons without Adele.

My running developed into a desire to compete, so I joined a running club, hoping to test myself as well as to form ties to other runners. I found the people there to be interesting and varied, not as superficial and more "real" than many of my co-workers.

My first attempt at achieving a formidable endurance goal occurred during the weekly running club competitions. I remember vividly that special Tuesday afternoon when the running club held its weekly time-trial run. My goal: to run the double-loop 5-mi course in less than 32 min.

From the onset of that time trial, I began to sense a pending personal victory as I felt the smooth flow of my legs pulling across the pavement. "Thirty-one fifty," the timer shouted at the 5-mi finish line. I had broken through my first fitness barrier! It was the first of many walls that would soon fall.

From then on, things began to fall into place rapidly. After being introduced to cross-training by a friend in January of 1986, I completed my first triathlon and won a trip to Hawaii to race in the Ironman Triathlon. By the following March, I had decided to become a professional triathlete.

Looking back at that first formidable fitness challenge of running the club time trial, I realize that it was the impetus that changed my whole outlook. I began to look at what I was eating, finally taking notice of the stuff I had been shoveling down my throat all those years. I asked myself questions like: What is the right thing to eat for an athlete? *The Complete Book of Running* and the *Vitamin Bible* replaced Harold Robbins on my bookshelf. I became interested in the intricacies of the human body—the variables, nutritional and otherwise, that affected how I ran.

Before embracing fitness, I felt as though my life was just a job description. Like so many people, I assumed a set role and struggled hard for approval from my peers. Whenever I felt despondent and unfulfilled, I convinced myself that I was doing exactly what I should be doing. But those nagging feelings kept coming back, and at times they would overwhelm me. I knew there had to be something more.

Exercise helped me realize that there are choices. The new opportunities and experiences fitness afforded me became evident and widened my perspective. With a fitter body, a sense of comfort and ease descended on me, and I came to realize that my physical fitness was closely tied to my self-esteem.

WHAT IS PEAK FITNESS?

Let's break down peak fitness into three basic aspects. Keep them in mind as you read through the coming chapters and put the advice, information, and exercise regimes into practice. Peak fitness is

- something you value (otherwise you wouldn't be reading this book);

- something you consider an achievement, whether in relation to personal health, improving your time or distance, controlling your weight, or winning a race; and

- usually fairly intense, not only in terms of physical effort but of mental exertion, resolve, and personal commitment.

VALUE

Exercise is an important part of your life—so important that you seek to achieve a level of fitness you've probably never attempted before. Perhaps you've caught some glimpses of it.

Maybe it was during the 90th mile of a 100-mi century bike ride, when you suddenly felt a rare burst of energy in your legs and passed 20 people before reaching the end. Maybe it was during your latest run, when in the last mile you had enough sustained power to climb that hill without letting up on your pace. Perhaps you've seen fleeting images of your athletic potential in the weight room, during an aerobics class, while in-line skating, or on a stair-climber.

Whatever situation caused you to believe—however slightly—that you could be much more of an athlete than you currently are, you see some value, some worth in working toward that goal.

ACHIEVEMENT

Peak fitness has everything to do with achievement, but there are as many ways to define *achievement* as there are types of running shoes (well, almost).

Achievement may be time-oriented; you may wish to finish a race or athletic event in a certain amount of time. Perhaps achievement is running a 10-km race in under the common 40-min threshold. Perhaps it means beating your best time on your favorite in-line skating course or in a race.

Achievement may simply mean completion. You may currently find it difficult to finish a weight room routine, a high-level aerobics class, or a masters swimming program workout.

And, of course, achievement may mean victory to you. You may have a goal such as winning a race overall, winning your age group overall, or beating your arch-rival, be it your brother, sister, girlfriend, best friend, or worst enemy.

INTENSITY

Intensity is a good word to describe many aspects of peak fitness.

A runner might seek a speed improvement by increasing the intensity of training on the track. An aerobics enthusiast might opt for a higher intensity workout, or a fitness enthusiast might design a more demanding workout regimen. The fitness level you aspire to may require a higher intensity on several levels.

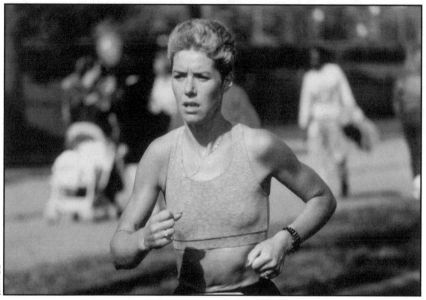

Peak fitness requires a high degree of intensity on a physical, mental, and emotional level.

PEAK COMPONENTS

Peak fitness is a term open to interpretation. Some might interpret it as total fitness, others as high cardiovascular fitness. But peak fitness doesn't just mean endurance. It means a degree of fitness that involves several major elements known by exercise physiologists as instrumental determinants of performance. These elements are

- cardiovascular conditioning,
- strength, and
- flexibility.

These three components make up the structure of a peak fitness exercise program and are dependent on each other in many ways. You can't do one and not the other without opening yourself up to vulnerabilities and weaknesses. You can't just concentrate on cardiovascular conditioning in endurance sports without giving some thought to strength training; by doing so you leave an area of imbalance in your exercise regimen that could cause you injury. By the same token, if you concentrate on strength training without paying heed to cardiovascular conditioning, you'll lack the endurance for almost any sustained activity.

These three components are illustrated in the Peak Fitness Triangle shown below. We'll learn more about the Peak Fitness Triangle later in this chapter, and we'll refer to it many times throughout the book.

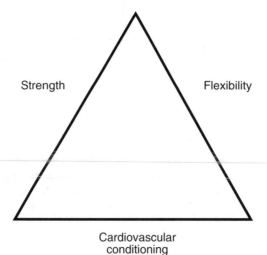

Strength

Flexibility

Cardiovascular
conditioning

Developing and maintaining flexibility at a young age can yield tremendous benefits down the line. In my early teens in South Africa, I was a fervent student of ballet. That's when I learned the value and benefits of flexibility, and later in life, I realized that the advantages of a flexible body carried over into endurance sports.

Flexibility, in particular, is a huge concern for athletes or for any woman over 40. It is one of the casualties of aging, thus older women have to work even harder on this side of the triangle. The older woman who continues to run or perform other aerobic activities with little regard for strength training and no stretching program may be fit enough to beat a man half her age at the local 10-km road race, but she is neglecting her health in a way that may lead to chronic arthritis or other similar conditions.

When considering the components of peak fitness, remember that a peak is something you attain only periodically. Peak fitness is composed of moments that are often brief—in reaching for the top of a mountain, the climber rarely spends much time at the summit. After reaching a peak, eventually you must begin the journey down. Then you plan for your next ascent, your next peak. To rise to ever-greater challenges, you have to continually change your approach up the mountain—go for another peak.

The concept is similar to the approach you might take to your career, or perhaps to working on a big project. You accomplish it and you feel good about it. But when it's over, it's time to start working for something else, to climb toward a new mountaintop.

Say you're a runner who is logging 20 mi a week and you set a goal of reaching 40 mi a week comfortably. You begin to build up your mileage gradually, taking care not to injure yourself by increasing it too quickly. Barring any mishap, within about 16 weeks you should have achieved your goal.

What do you do then? Retire from running and become a glutton? Not likely. You've reached what was once an elusive and lofty goal, and it has taken hard work, persistence, and self-discipline to achieve it.

Now, because you've caught that glimpse of your potential, you want to be even better. You're not content, and you know you can achieve more. You know because some weeks you feel like running 45 mi, and on some days you feel so strong the thought crosses your mind that you could run a marathon . . . and the following day, you start training for your first 26-miler.

For me, the training weeks preceding the Gatorade® Ironman World Championship Triathlon in Hawaii are when I am most fit. They are usually the three weeks in late summer when I'm in top shape for this race held in late October. I know when I'm at this level because I feel as though I could walk out my front door and comfortably train for 6 or 8 hr at a stretch.

WHAT YOU'LL GAIN FROM PEAK FITNESS

If you've been involved in fitness for awhile, I'm sure you already recognize the benefits of working toward challenging fitness goals, especially those that seem impossible. Besides the obvious physical benefits, you gain the mental toughness and focus that carry over into your everyday life.

Without consistent, recurring fitness challenges, your life is thrown out of balance. You feel run down. You lack energy. You lose the drive to take care of yourself. Even athletic people have gone through a period of staleness and inactivity, however brief. Chances are you remember when you were that way, and the memories aren't fond. Usually, when someone commits to a high level of fitness, exercise becomes a habit—a powerful, healthy habit.

You'll find numerous benefits to improving each of the three components of peak fitness. These benefits play a part in improving your mental and physical health, in increasing your ability to prevent injuries and disease, and in enhancing your ability to perform basic activities of daily living.

Your Mental and Physical Health

- **Your metabolic rate increases:** The rate at which you burn calories increases, making you less susceptible to weight gain and other weight-related health problems.

- **You delay aging:** As you get older, your metabolism tends to slow down. With a consistently demanding (not overdemanding) exercise program, you burn more calories in a day. Your body becomes more efficient, so instead of losing ground through the normal aging process, you're gaining ground.

- **You become more attractive:** A healthy and fit body shows—not just in the obvious improvements in physical appearance but in the attractive way you talk, walk, and carry yourself.

- **You reduce anxiety:** We've all heard about the calming, almost euphoric effects of the "runner's high." But feeling good after exercise doesn't just apply to runners. The psychological benefits of making exercise part of your lifestyle are numerous.

Injury and Disease Prevention

- Your body is more likely to be free of disease. The demands exercise places on the various bodily systems make the body stronger, more efficient, and less vulnerable to infection.

- As a result of greater flexibility and added strength, you may find that your propensity for injury is greatly decreased.

- There is less likelihood of falling prey to degenerative diseases. Particularly in women, osteoporosis, cancer, and other degenerative diseases have less chance of striking.

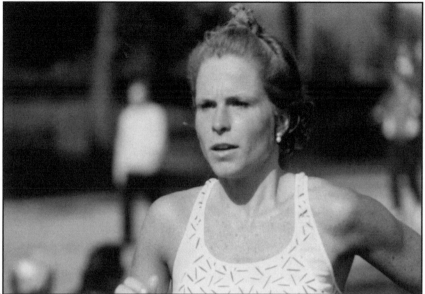

The "runner's high" doesn't just apply to marathoners, but to anyone who dedicates herself to peak fitness.

Improvement in Daily Living

- Daily physical chores are easier, and you're able to move your body in ways you previously thought impossible. You find it is much easier to lift things and to assume and maintain flexible body positions.

- You are sharper. Exercise—particularly vigorous, sustained exercise on a daily basis—increases your body temperature, boosting the amount of blood your heart pumps throughout your body. The result is more fuel (sugar) and oxygen going to your brain, which means you'll be more mentally focused for the normal demands of the day.

WOMEN'S ISSUES

Ironically, many of the same reasons that lead some women to seek peak fitness keep others from pursuing it. We've all heard someone say:

"I'll get bulky muscles if I strength train."

"Physical activity isn't feminine."

"It's just not healthy for women to pursue such strenuous activities."

If you dedicate yourself to safe and proper training in all three fitness areas—cardiovascular conditioning, strength, and flexibility—the previous statements will soon sound more like:

"My body looks attractive, firm, and toned because I strength train."

"I have more energy."

"I feel better and my body is much healthier."

In this section, I'll round out the various topics addressed in this book to help you achieve not only a peak fitness level but a correspondingly excellent health level and an appreciation and enjoyment of the process. By using this information, you will avoid the traps and behaviors (or nonbehaviors) that can lead to damaging or ignoring your health.

BEING FIT AND HEALTHY

The most important issue to consider on the path toward peak fitness is that you can be extremely fit yet not healthy. World-class athletes, in particular, have a hard time fully understanding this concept. In the competitive world of triathlon, for example, there are many women who have reached an impressive fitness level but have ignored their health to the point where illness and injury are commonplace.

The tendency to ignore one's health when striving for a high level of fitness can be blamed partly on the influence of our fast-paced society; our desire for instant gratification has ruined many a person's health. This mentality is apparent in the ads for instant diet plans and overnight fitness programs seen on television or on glossy magazine pages. People want instant fitness in the same way they drive to convenience stores hoping to win instant cash in the lottery. Impatience can easily pull you away from dealing with health issues in a rational, faithful way.

A frightening and all-too-common symptom of this approach to fitness is the rampant occurrence of anorexia and bulimia among female endurance athletes. We'll go into nutrition in greater detail in chapter 7, but the point I want to make here is that these dangerous conditions result from an ignorance of what being truly healthy is all about.

And not only do you endanger your health when you look at peak fitness purely from an instant, results-oriented point of view, you miss out on enjoying the process. For example, runners who force themselves out the door because they feel they *have to* run today, or *have to* go at this pace, or *have to* eat this way will experience little enjoyment; they will give little thought to the advantages of just running or to a simple appreciation of fitness. Even after positive results, such as a victory in a race, this lack of balance will often leave the athlete with a dwindling sense of gratification.

Remember, although getting there is important, the experience of getting there is just as important. When an outcome has finally been reached—whether successfully or not—disappointment or feelings of emptiness may stem from a lack of attention to the process.

MUSCLES ARE ATTRACTIVE

Many women grapple with the fear of developing a muscular appearance when they realize that strength training is a primary component of peak fitness. Much of the male population still adheres to society's view of the ideal woman as frail, fragile, and delicate. Even among women, there are a host of misconceptions and prejudices about weight training: working with weights is a masculine activity; women aren't designed for exercises that require strength; weight training will lessen sexual attractiveness.

Happily, though, there is growing consensus that a more defined female body is attractive and that a little more muscle is acceptable in women. And women are beginning to understand that true fitness is more than just being well-shaped. The horrible lesson of breast implants has shown women of the 90s that true fitness means having an attractive shape because you've sweated it out, you've done the exercise it takes, not just paid for the plastic surgery.

WORK TOWARD A BALANCED LIFESTYLE

More than ever, women are stressed out by the constant demands of family, career, and personal development. Although you may believe that striving for peak fitness will only add to these stressors, on the contrary, a well-planned workout schedule will help you become more efficient and give you more energy to tackle the other areas of your life.

Balance is also important in overcoming the negative stereotypes associated with the serious female athlete. Typically, the media has treated the Ironman triathlete, or any professional ultra-endurance athlete, as an oddity. Competitors are portrayed as obsessive, hard-as-nails, blister-bloodied Marine sergeant types teetering on the brink of self-destruction. That is just plain crazy.

Admittedly, that portrayal has put the sport on the map, but the reality is that my training is reasonable and sane and my lifestyle balanced and integrated. I do have hard days: long training rides of 100 mi or more when I long to be sitting on a La-Z-Boy recliner instead of my thin bicycle seat; killer swim workouts after which I walk away from the pool looking like a prune. Still, for the most part, my training regime is sensible, and I always allow myself enough rest and recovery time to heal mentally and physically.

I also find balance by making my training a social activity. There is a strong triathlon community in the small town of Encinitas, California, where I train with many of my competitors. In addition, I often run with friends who are not professional athletes—from my hairdresser to my agent.

Most professional athletes attempt to integrate their training with a well-rounded lifestyle. For any competitive athlete, a balanced training schedule and lifestyle makes for successful competition and a successful life.

WOMEN AND FITNESS

Regardless of what the term means to you, peak fitness is a concept that, until two decades ago, didn't pertain to women.

For many years, professional athletic associations were convinced that females could not handle the rigors of endurance sports. As recently as 1966, women were not allowed to participate in track distances of more than 1,000 m. It wasn't until 1981 that a 10,000-m track event for women was sanctioned by the International Amateur Athletic Federation. Amazingly, the women's marathon wasn't added to the Olympics until 1984.

Throughout these decades, women have been at the forefront of fitness. The increased opportunities for women in endurance sports in recent years have yielded many phenomenal performances, and world records for women have fallen faster than for men. For example, since 1955, the women's marathon record has improved by an astounding 61%, whereas men have shown only an 18% improvement.

Even in the sport of triathlon, where male participants outnumber females three to one, women are beginning to move to the forefront. In the Danskin Triathlon Series, a series of women-only races held throughout the country, an increasing number of first-time female triathletes swim, bike, and run on their way to peak fitness each year.

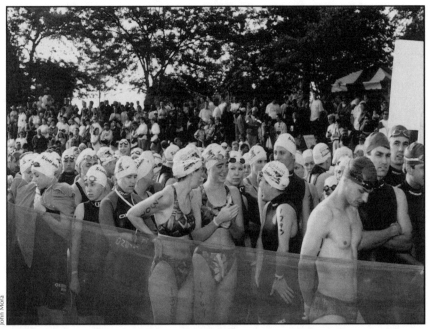

John Mora

Women have made tremendous athletic strides in recent years and the potential for greater achievements in sports is unlimited.

Overall, women have become more competitive in athletics. As role models, professional and age-group female athletes have shown the mainstream that you can run long distances and still have a normal menstrual cycle, that you can swim and be pregnant at the same time, and that there is no limit to what the female athlete can achieve.

Although women have traditionally been viewed as having far greater physical limitations than men, this theory is being proven wrong in road races, on the track, and in weight training rooms every day. It is also being disproven in exercise physiology labs.

An interesting debate has surfaced recently—supported by researchers at the University of California—that women are closing the gap on men in a few athletic arenas, most notably endurance sports. Look at ultramarathoner Ann Trason, who, in the 1990 24-hr ultramarathon world championship, ran more miles than anyone, including the men. In the sport of triathlon, my Ironman finish in 1988 was good enough for ninth place overall, and in the last 10 mi of the 26.2-mi run leg, I passed many top professional men (including my boyfriend, Paul Huddle, much to his dismay).

The male-female gap indeed seems to narrow in longer events. Some argue that women are better suited than men for endurance sports because of their higher body fat. Others say that the more patient and consistent pace of women in the first half of an endurance event allows them to excel overall.

But female athletes are closing the gender gap in shorter distance events as well. Consider Olympic swimmer Janet Evans, who finished the 400-m race 2 s faster than Mark Spitz's 1968 world record. Or how about speedskater Bonnie Blair, whose dizzying speed of 39.1 s over 500 m would have earned the gold in the men's event through 1972.

But the issues women face in taking on the challenge of peak fitness aren't really those of gender but of personal and individual commitment and achievement. What's important is that we now know that a high level of fitness is definitely attainable for the woman committed to a structured, intelligent training program.

Although peak fitness is a relatively new concept, it is growing in popularity, particularly among women. Thus, there is a need for up-to-date and specific fitness information for women. In the following chapters, I'll provide you with that information as well as share some personal experiences from my own quest for peak fitness.

Chapter 2

Investing in Peak Fitness

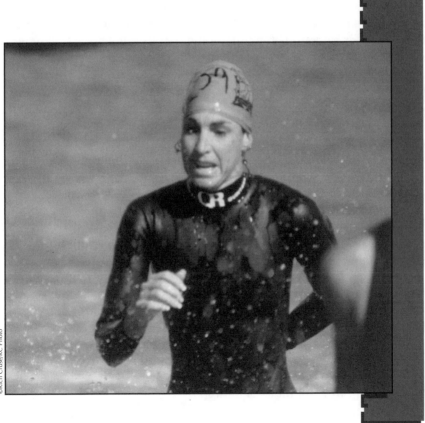

You *can* make substantial performance gains by devoting time to strength and flexibility training. Your gains may even be equal to—sometimes better than—the gains you'd make if you simply used that time for cardiovascular exercise (assuming you are already at a good to excellent cardiovascular fitness level).

If lack of competition isn't what's keeping you from paying as much attention as you should to strength training or flexibility, perhaps you're addicted to your favorite aerobic activity. Like a great number of runners addicted to that "runner's high," perhaps you feel uneasy or unproductive unless you're pounding the pavement with continuous 6-min miles, getting your heart rate into the 80% to 90% of maximum zone.

Peak fitness is a more balanced, long-term approach. If you're limited for time, that may mean cutting your track workout short by 20 min to do some stretching exercises, or perhaps cutting your 8-mi run down to 5 so you can spend some time doing triceps curls.

Changes do not have to occur overnight. Commitment, even a little at a time, will eventually get you where you want to go. If you have a hard time sacrificing 1 min from your normal cardiovascular routine, you must address your level of commitment. Are you willing to do what it takes to achieve peak fitness, even if it means leaving the comfort zone that you've established with your current exercise routine? It's simple really: to get different results you have to do things differently. And if you want to see some fitness improvements, you have to improve your fitness program.

If I seem to be harping on the importance of strength and flexibility training, it's simply because if you don't work with all three of the components of the Peak Fitness Triangle, your training program won't be complete.

Let's take a closer look at each of the three peak fitness components we discussed in the preceding chapter: cardiovascular conditioning, strength, and flexibility. Bear in mind that a thorough understanding of the role each component plays in your peak fitness regimen is vital to the success of your program. If you are prone to feigning interest in one or more of these areas of training, this attitude will make pushing beyond your current fitness performance levels 10 times harder and leave you more vulnerable to injury.

Once you've read through chapters 3, 4, and 5, which give more specific training information, you will better understand how each of the three components creates a powerful Peak Fitness Triangle. You also will see that a deficiency in any of the areas represented by the three sides can cause overall weakness.

CARDIOVASCULAR CONDITIONING

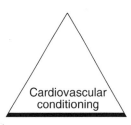

Cardiovascular conditioning

Cardiovascular conditioning forms the base of the Peak Fitness Triangle because it is the most fundamental measurement of fitness. Solid cardiovascular conditioning is essential to sustain training in the areas represented by the other two sides of the triangle: strength and flexibility. It also functions as a base because it's a solid foundation for any fitness program.

Cardiovascular conditioning simply means to condition the cardiovascular system to work more effectively and efficiently by supplying working muscles with needed oxygen. The human body is remarkable in its ability to help the lungs, heart, and circulatory system adapt to the increasing demands of a dynamic exercise program, activity that constantly pushes vital systems beyond their limits to improve performance.

Although the American College of Sports Medicine (ACSM) has recommended cardiovascular exercise for the general public since 1978, chances are that as a high-level fitness enthusiast, you're raising

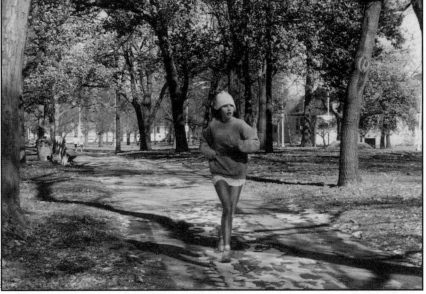

John Mora

The human body has a remarkable ability to adapt to exercise on a cardiovascular level. Activities such as running affect the lungs, heart, and circulatory system in a beneficial way.

your heart rate more than the recommended 20 min at a time, three times a week.

Although you may already be familiar with the performance benefits of cardiovascular conditioning, learning some basic (and easy-to-understand) exercise physiology may help solidify your commitment to a fitness-based lifestyle. Let's look at some of the fundamental changes that occur in the body as a result of cardiovascular exercise. These are only a small sampling of the changes and improvements that occur in your body every time you finish that 10-mi run or a 2-hr bike ride. Other significant transformations include stronger respiratory muscles, increased red blood cell count, and greater efficiency in carrying oxygen to other parts of the body.

STRONGER HEART

In essence, the heart becomes a stronger, more efficient muscle, resulting in increased stroke volume. In a well-conditioned athlete, the heart pumps as much as 20% to 30% more blood per beat than that of a sedentary person.

MORE EFFICIENT HEART

The heart resting rate of a high-level fitness athlete is usually 40 to 60 beats/min, much slower than the average of 70 to 80 (higher for sedentary people). This occurs for several reasons and is partially due to the heart pumping more blood per stroke.

BLOOD PRESSURE DECREASES

Although it may not be of concern to the high-level fitness enthusiast (unless you have a high-cholesterol diet), research has shown that blood pressure decreases as a healthy benefit of physical training.

A BETTER BLOOD DELIVERY SYSTEM

Continued and consistent endurance exercises carve larger and stronger blood pathways, which deliver more blood to working muscles. The network of capillaries increases, enabling muscles to receive more blood and leading to further improved performance.

AEROBIC AND ANAEROBIC: WHAT'S THE DIFFERENCE?

Most endurance athletes are familiar with the difference between long, slow distance workouts and interval or speed work, but are lost when it comes to understanding the distinction between aerobic and anaerobic exercise. Here's a simple explanation to help you understand the difference.

The word *aero* comes from the Latin word meaning "air." During aerobic exercise, you are working at an intensity level where the body is able to deliver oxygen to working muscles. Research has shown that aerobic conditioning occurs when you run at an effort of 65% to 90% of your maximum heart rate. Although you are working your muscles, ample air (oxygen) is being delivered to them.

Examples of aerobic exercise might include an easy run, a leisurely bicycle ride, any physical activity that is active, although not strenuous, for an extended period.

The prefix *an* means "without," so anaerobic literally means "without air." During anaerobic activity, the body's oxygen delivery system cannot keep up with exercise intensity. Your body begins to feel the effect of muscles without air (without oxygen) in the form of a burning sensation, called lactic acid buildup.

Some anaerobic activities include a finish line sprint, track workout intervals, and hill climbing. The anaerobic experience can also be felt in the weight room during a particularly intensive lifting session.

Although there is some overlap between aerobic and anaerobic exercise, and the thresholds vary with each individual, the anaerobic phenomenon will usually occur between 90% and 100% of your maximum heart rate (see figure on page 20).

STRENGTH

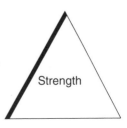

A good strength training program will enable you to make significant improvements in all areas of your body. The basic concept is to make you stronger and give you more overall balance.

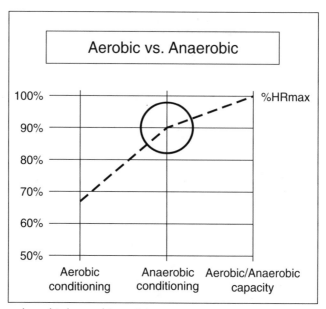

Heart rate and aerobic/anaerobic activity.

Adapted with permission from *Peak Running Performance* newsletter, January/February 1994, vol. 4, number 1, page 4. *Peak Running Performance* is a bimonthly newsletter that provides practical, up-to-date, expert, and scientific-based research information and performance-related ideas about running in an easy-to-use format for runners and their coaches. Write to PRP, Inc.; P.O. Box 3000; Dept. PRP; Denville, NJ 07834.

It's all about achieving maximum results with minimum effort. Or, if you want to look at it from another perspective, it's about making the most efficient use of energy. For example, if you bench press a certain amount when you begin, later you can lift more weight without any extra output of energy.

If you haven't paid much heed to strength training, you might find it more and more difficult to achieve a higher peak in your performances. Even if you're a top triathlete swimming 15,000 m, cycling 700 mi, and running 60 mi a week, there's a limit to how well you can perform by training in purely cardiovascular sports. My experience as a high-mileage junkie (more on this later) illustrates that even highly trained athletes reach a plateau and—in some cases—begin a downslide in performance. It can be a frustrating feeling. It seems as though you've hit a brick wall and you just can't get any better. You get to a point where you just seem to be sliding backward.

Runners often fall into this trap, believing that their performance will improve with greater mileage. If you're a runner, it doesn't matter how many miles you run or how many intervals you crank out. You will eventually reach the point where your performance can no longer be improved by purely cardiovascular means.

The same is true of almost any other endurance sport, whether it be cycling, swimming, in-line skating, or even race walking. Only so much can be achieved through increased mileage.

To reach your true potential, to get beyond performance barriers, to achieve peak fitness . . . you must look toward strength, toward increasing the energy output and efficiency of the muscles that power you through the repetitive exercise you are performing.

While some may argue that strength can be derived from a balanced cross-training program, doing solely aerobic training yields limited results. Although cross-training in several different cardiovascular activities can produce good muscular strength, it's very difficult to achieve balance using a purely multisport approach.

Imbalances will always show themselves. Cyclists have huge quadriceps but weak hamstrings. Swimmers have huge lats but weak legs. Runners have good lower body strength but poor upper body development.

Strength training is the balancer. It is a form of training that will compensate for the weaknesses and imbalances that are a natural result of using the same muscles over and over again in the same way.

FLEXIBILITY

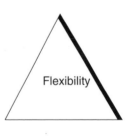

Flexibility training is one of the simplest ways to increase fitness, enhance the quality of daily life, and improve athletic performance. Anyone can do it, and it doesn't require additional financial resources or a high degree of energy. That's not to say you don't have to work at it—you do. But the long-term rewards far outweigh the initial investment.

Flexibility can help you increase your fitness level in a foundational way that affects almost every aspect of your exercise program. With flexibility, you can safely train for cardiovascular fitness, strength, and speed. Without flexibility, your range of motion in almost any activity is limited, and you become much more susceptible to injury.

With flexibility, daily living is enhanced because you stand taller, move more gracefully, and look better. You'll even have fewer musculoskeletal aches and pains caused by bad posture due to inflexibility.

Improved flexibility will improve your performance because it will increase your range of motion. Weight training increases the capacity of your muscles to be strong; flexibility training increases the range over which those same muscles can move. Strength and flexibility are tied together in this vital way. The increases in strength come at either end of your range of motion, as in running when you're working through your stride. The power comes from those improvements in range.

For example, running muscle might be 5 in. long, but with lactate buildup (during a strenuous run or during the latter stages of a marathon), the muscle shortens to only 3 in. long. If you can increase your running stride by half an inch, the overall effect of the increase in distance with each step will astound you. It can improve your marathon by minutes.

If you're a swimmer, increases in range of motion can have dramatic results. If you increase your range of motion in trunk rotation, for example, your stroke will improve. If your trunk rotation is a little better, your roll in the water is better, and thus your reach will help you go a little further with each stroke. Even with minimal improvement in trunk rotation, the effect can be great. It can add up to an inch per stroke, and when you apply that to a kilometer of swimming, it can take minutes off your best swimming time.

If you've never been a fan of stretching, either before or after exercise, prepare to commit to this activity on a whole new level. Stretching takes a lot of patience, but it can improve your performance.

You may consider flexibility training arduous and time-consuming. One reason many athletes are not motivated to stretch is that it's not a competitive activity. At least with weight training, even though you may not be part of a formal competition (unless you're a professional weightlifter), you can quantify the results. You can measure your progress much more easily and chart your improvement weekly or monthly, whether it's increased pounds you've lifted or an increase in repetitions, or both.

The lack of competition and measured progress are two reasons many athletes have poor or nonexistent stretching programs. Flexibility training is such a passive activity that, ultimately, the primary motivation must come from a firm commitment to a balanced program with a long-term vision of the benefits.

Not only do you have to be committed, you have to be consistent with your stretching program. If you begin a program, see some improvement, and then abandon your stretching for months, your gains will quickly be erased. When not pushed, your body will regress to its previous range of motion, negating all the effort and time you've put in.

In a nutshell, the components that make up the Peak Fitness Triangle enable you to get the most out of yourself. Peak fitness is about paying attention to the details of your body, details that are often overlooked or commonly considered the "stuff on the sidelines" that is relevant but not vital to performance. Reaching peak fitness may mean adjusting that perspective. To reach a high level of fitness, you have to bring some of these details to the forefront.

TALES FROM A MILEAGE JUNKIE

As an endurance athlete, it took me a long time to accept the importance of strength and flexibility training. As with many professional athletes, it came about as a result of a performance plateau.

I was running 40 mi a week and realized that I could handle 50. Pretty soon I was logging 70 mi a week, all the while maintaining my training in swimming and cycling. My entire fitness program was based on cardiovascular conditioning.

For a short time my running improved, but before long I leveled out, and eventually my performances began to decrease. I reasoned that I wasn't running enough miles, so I began to run 80 and sometimes 90 mi a week. Eventually my body broke down and I sustained a stress fracture in my ankle in June of 1993.

My doctor told me that I could return to cycling in 4 weeks and to running in 8 weeks, an eternity for a professional triathlete. I couldn't do any weight-bearing exercises, including walking, so the only viable aerobic activity was swimming.

This was devastating. The Gatorade® Ironman World Championship Triathlon in Hawaii is the one event I focus on all year, but without the chance to maintain and improve my cardiovascular fitness for this grueling 9-hr event, chances were slim that I would be able to compete.

I took some time to regroup and realized that all was not lost. I decided that I would do everything in my power to make my body more efficient, stronger, and more flexible. This meant refocusing my time and energy on strength training and stretching. For example, if I would normally be riding my bicycle for 2 hr in the morning, I committed myself to working instead on my upper body strength during that time. If I was supposed to run 1 hr, I'd spend it stretching. I was amazed that I could still spend 3-5 hr a day training without doing any running or cycling. A typical day during my period of recovery included

- 1 hr of swimming,
- 45 min of water running (non-weight-bearing),
- 90 min in the weight room, and
- 1 hr of stretching.

Within a few weeks, I was impressed with the significant improvements in my overall fitness and my renewed sense of well-being.

I was not allowed to do certain lower body exercises in the weight room, such as leg presses and squats. Again, I worked around that limitation and focused twice as hard on leg extensions and hamstring curls, two exercises that would not harm or hinder the injured area.

I took my usual stretching much more seriously and got involved in a special form of stretching called Pilates (which I'll talk about in chapter 3).

By July I was back on my bicycle, and in August, I put in my first running mile since the injury. Two months later, standing on the beach in Kona, I knew that—although I was lacking some endurance—my improvements in strength and flexibility made my body more efficient than those of many of my competitors.

What happened? I had my fastest swim and cycling leg ever. I was even on pace for my fastest run up to 15 mi, but because of my limited long-distance training, I began cramping. I had come too far, endured too much adversity to lose after leading for so long. Those last 11 mi were some of the hardest running I'd ever done, but I persevered and won.

When I look back and wonder what got me through, I realize that—besides a lot of heart—it was the strong, flexible muscles in my legs that kept me moving through those last difficult miles.

THE FINANCIAL INVESTMENT

Fortunately, your financial investment in flexibility training will be little or nothing, because stretching can be done virtually anywhere. If you do not have a soft surface on which to lie comfortably, you can purchase a foam-filled exercise mat at any sporting goods store for less than $50.

As for strength training, weight equipment can be pretty pricey: from $400 for a simple weight bench, barbell, and dumbbells setup to $4,000 and up for a multistation weight machine. Many of the strength training exercises that are illustrated in chapter 4 can be performed at home with a simple weight bench setup, but some of the exercises require the use of expensive weight training machines.

HEALTH CLUBS

I recommend joining a health club if it's an option where you live. Consider one that has a variety of strength training equipment as well as a free weight room. Of course, if you are a triathlete or swimmer, make sure the club has a clean swimming pool with designated lanes for lap swimming. Although you may have to pay an initial membership fee that will seem expensive, if you use the facilities consistently, the price will be worth it.

Even if you are a member of a well-equipped health club, you may want to have some relatively inexpensive strength training equipment around the house for convenience. As mentioned earlier, a weight bench, dumbbells, and a barbell with a few weights can be purchased for a few hundred dollars.

You'll also need some strength training equipment when you travel. (No, you won't have to pack your dumbbells.) In chapter 4, we'll discuss surgical tubing, which is a handy way to strength train on the road for less than $10.

SPORTS EQUIPMENT

In terms of the specific equipment used in your sport, your financial investment should be directly proportional to your time commitment. You can finish an Ironman with an old 10-speed bomber, but if you want performance, you have to take your equipment to a higher level.

Every bolt, every component, the frame material, the wheels, and the accessories on my bicycle have all been chosen for winning performance. Like a race car pit crew, the expert staff at my local shop has helped me to build the most aerodynamic, efficient, and lightest bike possible.

Of course, my bicycle didn't come cheap, but I'm a professional with thousands of dollars of sponsorship and prize money on the line with every race. If you're not a professional, you have to gauge how important equipment is and how much you're able and willing to spend. If you're serious about what you're doing, you can afford it, and you feel the equipment will significantly help you, then go for it.

If you haven't made some basic equipment purchases, your first step should be to visit a local shop that specializes in your sport. But in your initial stages, be careful not to get swept up in a purchasing frenzy that leaves you with no money to pay the mortgage.

TRIATHLON EQUIPMENT

In the sport of triathlon, equipment is a major issue. Triathletes have introduced new technology into the traditional world of cycling, providing such innovations as aerodynamic handlebars, as well as advances in disk wheels, helmets, and frame designs and materials. Other innovations include wetsuits, swimming aids, and running shoes.

Although equipment is important in a technical sport such as triathlon, don't fall into the trap of overemphasizing equipment. Don't let a preoccupation with things overshadow the time, energy, and resources you put into making your engine (your body) more efficient and stronger.

Nevertheless, for the serious triathlete, there are a few equipment investments that are essential. In the next section, I'll discuss three major triathlon equipment upgrades you may want to consider because of their proven performance benefits.

Wetsuits

Many triathletes—even the veterans—find open-water swimming unnerving. Indeed, the statistics show most triathletes come from a running rather than a swimming background. The Triathlon Federation/USA estimates that more than 50% of triathletes began their athletic careers as runners, which explains why wetsuits are so popular among triathletes.

What is so great about wetsuits? Do you really need to shell out several hundred bucks for one? An indication of their usefulness is that at your next triathlon, you may be the only one standing on the beach in just your swimsuit.

The benefits of swimming with a wetsuit depend on numerous factors, such as percentage of body fat, stroke efficiency, body temperature, and a host of other variables. However, there are four areas of consistent return on a wetsuit investment for the serious triathlete interested in improving swim times:

- Improved buoyancy
- Greater warmth in cold temperatures
- Energy conservation
- Greater speed

The most important consideration when shopping for a wetsuit is fit. The key? Take your time and get it right. Until you find a wetsuit that fits you like a second skin, don't be satisfied with anything less. Here are five practical tips on purchasing and using a wetsuit:

- Choose a wetsuit design based on where you intend to do most of your swimming. If you swim in very cold water, a full-length

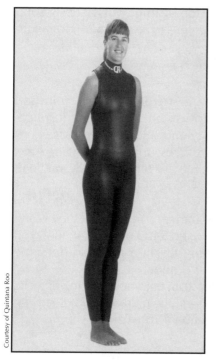

Courtesy of Quintana Roo

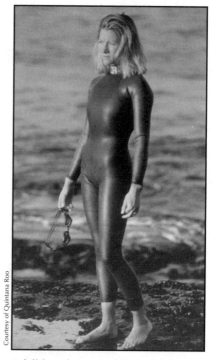

Courtesy of Quintana Roo

Sleeveless wetsuits allow upper body mobility while providing warmth, buoyancy, and energy conservation.

A full-length wetsuit is best if you swim in very cold open water. Although a full-length wetsuit can take a little longer to get off, it is unsurpassed in providing warmth.

wetsuit is best. Sleeveless designs are good for most situations, and the mini-wetsuit or "Quickjohn" design is best when temperature is not a factor.

- Pay close attention to how the wetsuit fits in the armholes (for sleeveless designs), neck area, and ankles. These are the locations where excess water is most likely to enter.

- The fit should be tight, but not so tight that you can't breathe normally or your motion is constricted.

- Once you buy your wetsuit, practice in open water before a race. You'll find that the added buoyancy may change your style, and some subtle adjustments will come with practice.

- If you're a triathlete, practice removing your wetsuit immediately following an open-water swim. This will help you speed up the tricky transition between swimming and cycling.

Wetsuits start at a little more than $100 for the mini-wetsuit design and range from $150-$200 for sleeveless designs to around $250 for a full-length wetsuit.

Aerodynamic Wheels

Bicycle equipment is undoubtedly the largest expense for the multisport athlete or serious cyclist, but the lofty prices are not without justification. An astounding level of technology and scientific expertise goes into designing bicycle components and accessories. Because the sport is so technical, the benefits to the athlete are tangible and practical, more so than with other sports.

For example, if you owned a pair of $50 shoes, you could spend $100 more on the best pair of running shoes money can buy, but they won't make you run any faster. But if you invested $400 in a disk wheel, you would significantly reduce your cycling leg in a triathlon. In some cases, the reduction can be as much as 5 min.

Assuming that you already own (at least) an entry-level racing bicycle, purchasing a set of aerodynamic wheels can help bring your "steed" up to speed. There are four types of production aerodynamic wheels:

- Disk wheels
- Three-spoked wheels
- Four-spoked wheels
- Deep-rim wheels

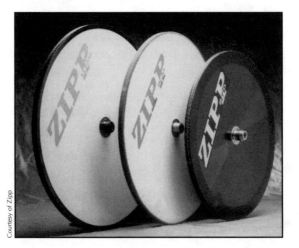

Courtesy of Zipp

Wind tunnel tests show that disk wheels, though not as effective in a crosswind, are still the most aerodynamic wheels for head-on winds.

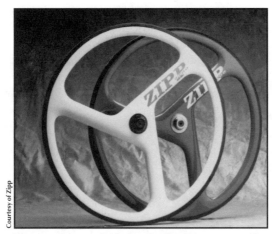

Courtesy of Zipp

Three- or four-spoked wheels offer the serious cyclist versatility and an aerodynamic advantage.

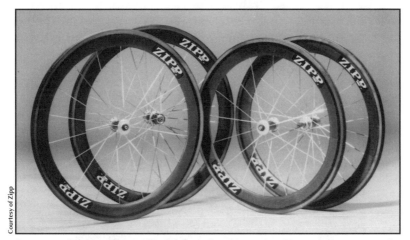

Courtesy of Zipp

Because of their greater affordability, deep-rim wheels are the most popular choice of triathletes.

Go to a bicycle dealer who specializes in triathlon or time-trial bicycles to get a better idea of the differences and advantages of each type of aerodynamic production wheel.

Another good option that many competitive road racers choose is purchasing a set of custom-built wheels. You can have a professional wheelbuilder at a pro bike shop tailor a wheel to your specifications. Some of the specifications might include an ultra-lightweight aerodynamic rim or bladed spokes that slice through the wind better.

Most disk wheels, three-spoked, and four-spoked wheels will cost you at least $500, with prices ranging all the way up to $800. Deep-rim wheels are slightly more economical, ranging from $300 to $500 (depending on the rim material, spokes, and hub).

Whether you decide to upgrade your standard spoked wheels with a custom-built wheel or an aerodynamic one, either will improve your performance. And depending on how heavy your current wheels are, they will decrease the weight of your bicycle noticeably, which brings us to the next upgrade.

Lightweight Replacement Parts

Nowadays, a wide selection of lightweight stems, seat posts, hubs, spokes, rims, bottom brackets, cranks, and cogs made of steel, titanium, aluminum, carbon fiber, and metal matrix are available to triathletes looking to lighten the load of their bicycles. Are these ultralight replacement parts worth the lofty prices you'll pay? Ultimately, you have to decide how serious you want to be about this bicycle stuff, but lightweight replacement parts can significantly decrease total bicycle weight, making it easier for you to climb on steep ascents and enabling you to accelerate much faster out of a turn on flat courses.

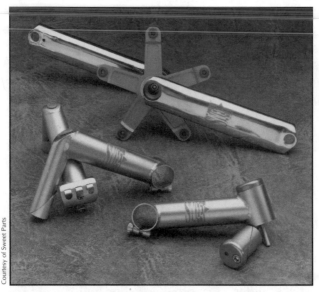

Courtesy of Sweet Parts

Lightweight replacement parts, such as the crankset/bottom bracket combination and stems pictured here, can significantly reduce weight on your bicycle for greater acceleration and lighter climbs.

How much weight can you save? As much as 50%. For example, a titanium cog, one of the heaviest component parts, is 50% lighter than cogs made of standard metal alloys.

Although lightweight replacement parts are expensive, the good news is that you don't have to replace all your parts at once. You can opt to replace your standard seat post with a titanium seat post one month, and with next month's paycheck, replace your standard spokes with ones made of lightweight carbon fiber.

The price ranges of lightweight replacement parts vary according to the specific part and material used. Again, if you're interested in lightening up your bike, consult with a bicycle dealer specializing in high-performance bicycles and bicycle components.

THE SOCIAL INVESTMENT

Unless you're a certified hermit, you should consider joining organizations and group workouts in your sport(s). There may be a fee to join, but the costs are usually minimal compared to the benefits of friendship and healthy competition. One important benefit of joining a group is the knowledge you'll gain from coaches and colleagues who are more familiar with the techniques, training methods, and nutrition related to your sports. In chapter 8, when I outline my training schedule, you'll see that group workouts are a major ingredient in my overall plan.

In some sports, such as cycling, the group workout can be your most fun—and challenging—session of the week.

Cycling in a pack can be a harrowing, nerve-racking experience if you're not used to riding in proximity to other riders. Just turning a corner with a cyclist on each side of you, 2 in. away, is enough to make you want to hit your brakes and turn around halfway into the ride (although I wouldn't recommend it—there would probably be someone 2 in. behind you who wouldn't appreciate that move). Which is precisely why—if you want to be serious about cycling or triathlon—you need to be there. Cycling is a very technical sport, and triathletes, in particular, tend to lack these skills.

The most demanding cycling workout on my weekly training schedule is the "Wednesday Ride" in the North County of San Diego. This group ride has been a triathlon tradition since 1985. Tens of triathletes and cyclists show up at a local bike shop, and from there we ride up the coast at an easy warm-up pace. More cyclists join us as we head toward the Camp Pendleton Military Base. Once onto the base, the pace picks up, and pretty soon it feels like we've been transported to the Tour de France. Once through the base, we crank out a lot of fast and furious miles racing on an old highway that is closed to traffic.

As you can imagine, it is a grueling, highly competitive, and aggressive 75 mi. (The motto of the ride is "Every man and woman for himself.") Cyclists with a variety of ability levels show up, but obviously the professional triathletes and international cycling pros dominate the lead group. This high level of cycling talent, as well as the dizzying speeds that can be reached in a large cycling group, make this an outstanding workout, something I would not be able to achieve on my own.

If you're interested in this type of workout, most bicycle shops conduct group rides or know of local cycling clubs that work out on a weekly basis.

Group running workouts provide similar benefits, although running isn't nearly as technical as cycling. For longer runs, a group workout can help ease the boredom, or at least allow you to share it with someone else. For those who want to improve their running performance, track workouts can reduce your running times significantly (although I'd recommend having a coach conduct interval sessions). Most local running clubs conduct group runs or track workouts or can point you in the right direction.

My weekly running group sessions are called the "Tuesday Run," another tradition for the triathlon community of Southern California. Every Tuesday at about 7:30 a.m., 50 or so runners and triathletes gather at the Rancho Sante Fe Country Club to put in about 12 mi of slightly hilly trail and flat golf course running. After 8 mi of hilly trail running, we begin a form of interval training on flat golf course terrain, putting in surges of speed or "pick-ups" that last about 2-3 min, with a 2-min recovery. Immediately following the golf course is the "Canyon Trail," a terribly steep hill about a mile long. (This is the acid test for fitness in our group and a nightmare for anyone who has gone too hard on the flats. I've seen many a fit athlete walking up this hill.)

If you're tired of running alone or need a new challenge, local running shops or clubs are your best bet to join a local "fun run" or track workout.

Admittedly, the rigidity of swimming can make going to the health club a dreadful experience. A human being can only take so much swimming . . . back and forth, back and forth . . . before developing "blue line fever." Although you might think that swimming is one sport you have to do alone, there are many organized swim group workouts and programs that will help push you to greater speeds. Working out with a masters swimming group or participating in swimming competitions can make swimming an invigorating experience.

I participate in the Carlsbad Masters Swim Program in the North County of San Diego, where I do all my pool swimming. Every Monday and Friday at 6:00 a.m. and every Wednesday at noon, I swim with other triathletes or masters swimmers.

The advantage of participating in a masters swim program is that each workout has a definite purpose and structure. Coaches are also there to help with my stroke technique. Because each of us at the Carlsbad workout has to share a lane (often with two or more people) I'm always pushed to maintain a reasonably fast pace to avoid holding up the swimmer behind me. If you don't find the experience too intimidating, swimming "circles" in a large group can push you harder and teach you to pace yourself through the entire session, a valuable lesson for racing.

Local colleges and health clubs are good places to begin your search for a swimming program.

Strength training and other exercises performed at a health club offer the fitness enthusiast an excellent chance for social interaction. Although the temptation is to become too engrossed in socializing (some health clubs are like singles bars), as long as the workout is accomplished, it helps to have people around to motivate you and push you harder.

Aerobics is an excellent example of the benefits of group motivation. Only a group environment, headed by a qualified and motivating instructor with inspiring music, can provide the excitement and momentum needed for a challenging workout.

I've only covered swimming, biking, running, strength training, and aerobics, but most communities have group workouts in almost every popular sport or exercise activity. Your best bet is to contact sporting goods stores or shops specializing in your activity; they should be able to put you in touch with local contacts. If you can't find information on group workouts through these sources, try contacting a national organization, which you can locate through your local library.

THE INTELLECTUAL INVESTMENT

Depending on how serious you are about your fitness goals, you need to invest a certain amount of time in obtaining valuable sport-specific knowledge. For example, if you want to become a better cyclist, you should become intimately familiar with the parts of your bicycle, perhaps studying how gearing ratios can affect your performance. If you want to improve your marathon time, you'd be well-advised to study the eating habits of top marathoners and the latest research on sports nutrition.

No longer is athletics simply an arena of physical prowess—any professional athlete who believes this is living in a dream world. Modern endurance athletes must be knowledgeable in several scientific and mechanical subjects related to their sport. The most fundamental areas of study include exercise physiology, sports psychology, sports nutrition, biomechanics, equipment maintenance and function, and aerodynamic theory.

You've heard it said that knowledge is power. In the world of professional athletics, that is literally true. It can mean the difference between a mediocre performance and a world record.

But you don't have to embark on a 4-year college course to gain knowledge. Countless resources are available to you at the local library or bookstore. Subscribe to magazines dedicated to the sport(s) in which you want to improve. If you're a cyclist, many local shops offer classes on bicycle maintenance. Commit yourself to learning one new thing about your sport each week or to reading one new book a month.

THE TIME INVESTMENT

Finding time to increase your fitness level can be difficult. However, in most cases, it is possible to attain a reasonably good fitness level with a limited daily routine, as long as you are realistic about your goals.

For example, if you are a runner who has just 20 min a day to exercise, you should be training for no more than a 5-km road race. But if you're training for an Ironman Triathlon, you're going to have to train much more, perhaps 1 to 3 hr a day during the week and 2 to 6 hr on weekends.

For the die-hard endurance athlete, the temptation is to ignore the other two sides of the Peak Fitness Triangle when time is limited. We'll explore workout structures and training schedules in chapter 8, but it's vital for you to realize from the beginning that you must set aside a certain amount of time to increase your strength and flexibility.

THE EMOTIONAL INVESTMENT

The emotional investment, more than any other, is absolutely essential to attaining peak fitness. What does the term *emotional investment* mean? Primarily, it means understanding and using the underlying emotional motivation that is at the root of your quest for peak fitness.

Most New Year's resolution exercise routines fail miserably for lack of this kind of vision. Although the health clubs are packed in January, it's easy to find a parking space in June. Why? Because most people don't take the time to document their motivation. They may spend an evening writing up a schedule or a goal chart, which they proudly post on their refrigerator door for all to see, but they don't bother to examine and write down their reasons for embarking on this new exercise regime.

Goals are important—extremely important—but if you don't have a clear idea of why you are setting those goals, your motivational level will more than likely decrease with each passing day, making you more and more susceptible to failure.

If you've made all the other investments, take the time to document—whether in a diary, computer journal, or exercise log—your true emotional motivation in striving for peak fitness. Keep it someplace where you will see it constantly, perhaps next to your schedule or goal chart on the refrigerator door.

Central to my success has been my long-standing emotional motivation to use endurance sports as a means of personal development and fulfillment. Early in my triathlon career, I decided to devote my life to learning more about my body and to finding new and creative ways of training and racing and teaching them to others. Every day I am motivated by a desire for complete health and a high level of fitness. I am moved by an internal sense of accomplishment that comes from my continual quest to fulfill my potential.

The question I'm asked most frequently is, "How can you train day after day after day without getting tired of it?" The answer is that my emotional investment in peak fitness has given me an almost inexplicable sense of enjoyment (which most people still don't understand). This motivation is what enables me to ride a bicycle for 5 hr one day, then go out and run an hour and a half the next.

I do it gladly.

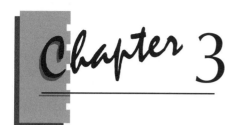

Chapter 3

Flexibility Training

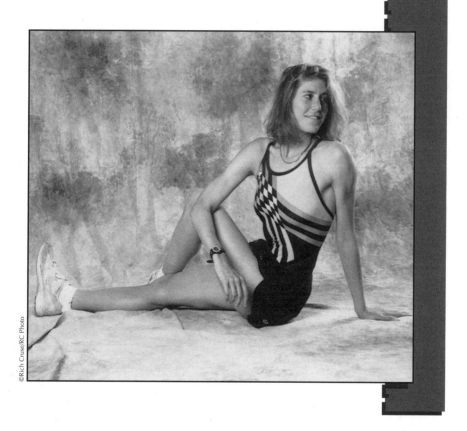

In 1993 I got a call from Dr. Morris Mann, a flexibility coach who specializes in stretching techniques for improved performance. He told me how increased flexibility could help me achieve a full range of motion and increase my biomechanical efficiency in swimming, cycling, and running.

It was clear from our conversation that he knew what he was talking about. He'd worked with other professional athletes and had achieved measurable improvements in performance, most notably in Olympic gold medalist Pablo Morales and the Stanford University swim team. From the tone of Dr. Mann's voice, I could tell he was passionate about flexibility training and professional sports and excited about the possibility of working with me.

Everything he said made sense, but at the time, I was neither ready nor willing to commit to the time and the effort he proposed. As mentioned in chapter 1, I've been a proponent of stretching since the days I trained as a ballet dancer. Still, I'd always looked at stretching as more of a necessity than a performance enhancer. So, essentially, I put him off.

A few months later, during a visit to the San Diego area, Dr. Mann met with Ironman champion Mark Allen and me. He convinced us of the importance of stretching and persuaded us to commit to stretching on a whole new level.

Several months later came my stress fracture injury. Because of all the time spent and knowledge accummulated on stretching before the injury, I was able to put it to good use during my recovery. The flexibility training techniques I learned and used during the painstaking months of rehabilitation were a major factor in my successful comeback.

I hope there is no doubt that the three components needed to reach peak fitness are cardiovascular conditioning, strength, and flexibility. Of these three, flexibility is the component that is lost most rapidly with age. Strength and endurance from cardiovascular conditioning seem to be factors that are much more dependent on other physiological factors.

Does this mean that maintaining, or even increasing, flexibility is a losing battle because we're aging every day of our lives? Perhaps, if you take a passive role by not participating in a consistent flexibility training program. But if you take responsibility for your body, the aging factor can be virtually negated, and in most cases, flexibility can be increased for measurable performance gains.

WHAT IS FLEXIBILITY?

Flexibility training is an important part of athletics, no matter what your sport. Yet, most athletes have only a cursory understanding of the mechanics and anatomy behind the flexibility of joints. So bear with the technical jargon; later on, as you participate in the flexibility exercises, this knowledge will help you to better understand the purpose of stretching.

THE SCIENCE OF FLEXIBILITY

In a broader sense, flexibility means *being capable of responding to change*. When applied to exercise physiology, this translates into joint mobility, or the ability of a joint to move freely in a normal, functional direction.

There are many variables that affect joint mobility, including the following:

- The structure of the joint itself
- The connective tissue elasticity within the muscles, tendons, and skin surrounding a joint
- Neuromuscular coordination

Naturally, flexibility is determined primarily by the supporting connective tissue that links the muscles and tendons to bones. Collagen, a fibrous protein that strengthens and supports the connective tissue in the body, is an integral component of this system. Flexibility is *not* determined by muscle size and stiffness. It is instead a function of the collagen, which is a product of genetics and environmental conditions.

The hard fact is that flexibility is decreased at the rate of 1%-2% a year, starting from the age of 19. Don't let that discourage you, though. Once again, taking an active role in helping your body to become more flexible requires time and commitment to a program. A consistent flexibility training program can minimize the factors that limit your range of motion with age.

THE PSYCHOLOGY OF STRETCHING

If we were to apply the definition of flexibility to the mind, descriptions such as "pliable" and "capable of responding or conforming to change or new situations" would seem appropriate. In many ways, flexibility begins with the mind, not the body.

As a physiological rule, the younger a person is, the more flexible and pliable their joints. However, there are many young people who are physically inflexible and many older people who have the flexibility of a young person.

The process of becoming more flexible should first center on who you are at present and where and how you intend to "move" in the future. The flexibility of our minds is like energy; we cannot measure it, but it creates the force that drives our physical body. This energy can drive us to pursue physical flexibility, which is more tangible and quantifiable.

People who have actively embraced a flexibility training program and are physically very flexible, especially older people, tend to be less willing to accept the perceived or prescribed limits of physiology. They are better able to accept those things that are permanent yet still believe in the existence of something they can't see, such as their goal of increased flexibility.

Try to keep an open (flexible) mind if all this sounds very "New Age" to you. Reality is also accepting that on the physical level, stretching and committing to improving flexibility takes time and hard work. It also requires a lot of faith in yourself and in your body's ability to improve. You won't see gratification instantly, but if you stick to a consistent flexibility training program, you will see improvement over a period of time.

It is also useful to look at your approach to increasing flexibility as a whole. As you learn and integrate the forthcoming stretches into your weekly program, try not to look at each individual exercise as only involving one particular muscle or region of the body. The body is an intricate system, with each muscle, each ligament, each cell affecting the entire system in subtle ways we've only begun to understand.

Among athletes, especially with regard to injury, an attitude of specialization is far too rampant. If a runner has a knee problem, all too often the tendency is to treat the knee without regard to other parts of the body that might be causing the damage. The problem could easily be the result of a back problem or a foot imbalance, both common causes of knee injuries. If a cyclist has a back problem, the root of the injury will more than likely be the position of her legs on the bike, or possibly the position of her foot on the pedal.

The same applies to flexibility. Every muscle is part of the whole body; when the range of motion of one joint is increased, it affects the entire system.

Familiarity breeds complacency, and a typical mistake when starting a stretching regimen is to look upon it solely as a form of relaxation, something that would be beneficial, perhaps, but certainly not a necessity. As a result, the inspired and focused workouts are devoted to intervals on the track or to the sprint at the end of a group ride. Stretching, if done at all, is often just an afterthought.

Although some stretching aids have become available in recent years, no external device will help you significantly increase your flexibility as much as a positive attitude. And if you've felt limited by your age or body type, be assured that there is nothing external that can stop you either. Ultimately, your body will go where your mind leads. Your best piece of equipment is internal—an inspired, focused, and committed attitude toward stretching.

THE STRETCHING HABIT

Because I'm such a fervent competitor, committing the time and energy to stretching was a major mental adjustment. Before my involvement with Dr. Morris Mann, I viewed stretching mainly as a means of relaxation. The necessary attitudinal shift I had to make was to view stretching as a workout in itself, or at the very least, as a significant component of my training.

The first thing I did was set aside a certain time of day for my stretching routine, usually after an aerobic activity like running. But even when I did that, I found myself tempted to "blow it off" and head for the shower. It took a lot of self-discipline, but I found that keeping the benefits of these exercises at the forefront of my thinking was crucial.

Music also helped motivate me to get into the stretching habit. I would put on my favorite CD, and the music would elevate my energy levels, making it easier to begin the workout. Once I had performed two or three stretches, the rest seemed easy and enjoyable.

Stretching has become such an established part of my routine that I don't hesitate at all to begin. In my schedule, stretching holds the status of an individual workout. It's taken me a long time, but with a little self-discipline, some motivating music, and a lot of persistence, I've successfully acquired the stretching habit.

THE BENEFITS

In the next few sections, perhaps the real challenge won't be to learn the exercises but to adopt a new approach toward stretching and improving your flexibility. The fact is that it's hard work, although perhaps a different kind of work than you may be used to. It is, in great part, a mental challenge that dares you to make a commitment and become responsible for a critical component of fitness you may have relegated to the sidelines in the past. A quick review of the benefits derived from greater flexibility might help you look at stretching in a whole new way.

IMPROVING PERFORMANCE

Perhaps the most attractive benefit of stretching is improved physical performance for the athlete. The more flexible a joint, the greater its ability to move through a wider range of motion and thus function more efficiently. Recent research at the Human Performance Laboratory at Boise State University showed that 20 min of stretching, three times a week, can increase your range of motion by 30%.

More specifically, stretching increases the ability of muscle fibers to generate force despite accumulation of lactic acid. Because muscle fibers act by contracting, the longer they are to begin with, the more they are able to contract. Optimum flexibility is accomplished when normal muscle fiber is as long as possible, so that when it inevitably shortens with the introduction of lactic acid into the system—as during anaerobic exercise or prolonged aerobic exercise—it is still able to function efficiently.

PREVENTING INJURY

Exercise physiologists generally agree that greater flexibility, and hence greater range of motion, makes people less likely to injure themselves.

The majority of traumatic muscular injuries occur when an athlete pushes a joint beyond its normal range of motion. The nerves that drive working muscles and give them their "memory" are surrounded by a sheath of muscle. If the sheath surrounding the nerve is elongated through stretches, the "memory" of the muscles is adapted to correspond with this greater range of motion, so when you push your joints beyond their normal range of motion, your muscles are able to react effectively, reducing the likelihood of injury.

IMPROVING COORDINATION

Greater flexibility increases neuromuscular coordination. It has been shown that the speed of nerve impulses is enhanced with stretching. The central nervous system becomes more sensitive to the physical demands placed on it, so opposing muscle groups work in a more coordinated way.

PROMOTING JOINT ELASTICITY

There is greater circulation to the joints. Stretching increases the temperature of the tissue, which in turn increases the blood and nutrients supplied to the joint structure. This process promotes greater elasticity in the surrounding tissue.

ENHANCING POSTURE AND MOVEMENT

Muscular balance and kinesthetic awareness are improved. Stretching helps realign soft tissue structures that may have less-than-optimum development due to normal biomechanical wear and poor posture. This realigning of tissue structure helps promote and maintain good posture and healthy movement in daily activities and athletics.

DECREASING BACK PAIN

The incidence of lower back pain decreases in individuals who participate in a regular flexibility training program. The American Council on Exercise indicates that there is strong clinical evidence to show that lumbar-pelvic flexibility, including hamstrings, hip flexors, and muscles attaching to the pelvis, is critical in decreasing stress to the lumbar spine.

RELIEVING MUSCLE TENSION

Stretching can relieve muscle tension. When muscles are tense for long periods of time (as during long endurance activities), the flow of oxygen to these muscles can be cut off. The result is a buildup of lactic acid in tissues, causing fatigue and muscle tightness or knotting. Stretching can help break up those muscle knots and release lactic acid into the bloodstream.

STATIC STRETCHING TECHNIQUE

There are about as many stretching techniques for athletes as there are sports drinks. The optimum stretching technique has long been—and probably will continue to be—a matter of controversy. The type of stretching technique recommended in this book is called static stretching. It is a conservative technique—traditionally accepted as safe and effective—that involves a gradual elongation through a full range of motion. In more basic terms, it means consistently trying to stretch a given area to a point of slight discomfort.

This type of stretching has been found to produce long-term gains that are maintained in people who practice consistently. This is because static stretching is low-intensity and imposes less microtrauma to the tissue, resulting in better flexibility without the danger that exists with more radical (and more painful) stretching techniques.

STRETCHING PRINCIPLES

The following are some basic principles to consider when starting and executing a static stretching program.

- Take off your shoes and socks before you begin and wear clothing that allows freedom of movement.

- If you follow a stretching program consistently over several months, you will experience excellent flexibility benefits. Three sessions a week will result in a definite improvement. Four sessions a week will show a significant improvement. Five sessions a week will show a more permanent improvement, even if you reduce the frequency for some time after that.

  A Swedish study found that once optimal flexibility had been attained, stretching just one or two times a week would maintain those gains. However, the study also found that if stretching was continued three to five times per week, the range of motion was further improved. So you can literally choose how far you want to go.

- Regardless of how good you are or how addicted you may become to stretching, always take one day off a week.

- Breathe through your nose. The reason for doing so is that your breath becomes an inhibitor that protects you from going too far beyond your current range of motion. If you reach a point in the stretch where you are no longer able to breathe through your nose, you have probably gone too far.

  In addition, by taking long, slow, deep breaths throughout both the inhalation and exhalation, you are better able to move into the stretch in a controlled way.

Breathing through your nose is usually more controlled than breathing through your mouth. Hence the stretching done in conjunction with your breathing will be more controlled.

- Under no circumstances should you bounce during the stretches. This only increases the risk of excessive microtears in the muscles.

- There will always be discomfort when you extend into some of the stretches. The key is to be careful but persistent. Work into each movement slowly, accessing the stretch. When you cannot extend any further, stop. This is the point at which your body needs to work, at least for now. This point will be different on different days, particularly as you become more flexible and accomplished at doing the exercises.

- Stretches can feel different each day. Some days are easier than others, depending on the other activities you have been doing. In addition, muscles are made up mainly of water, so if you are dehydrated, it will decrease your flexibility. Perform the stretches on an empty stomach to prevent cramping.

- Elevated tissue temperature increases range of motion. The normal temperature of a muscle at rest is 98°F. After aerobic exercise, the temperature is elevated to about 102°F. This makes the muscle more pliable and less likely to tear. Therefore, you should perform more rigorous stretches after an aerobic workout because there will be maximum gains in range of motion.

- Concentrate on proper alignment in each stretch to achieve maximum results in the specific muscle group you're working on. Proper alignment promotes a good "relationship" between the muscles and joints, fostering cleaner and more efficient lines of movement. This will also help you overcome any biomechanical problems you might have due to poor technique or postural imbalances.

- Once you have gradually and slowly moved into the stretch, hold it for 15-30 s or 5-10 breaths, whichever works better for you. As you become more familiar with the stretches and want to work them a little more, hold them into the 30-s or 10-breath range.

STRETCHING EXERCISES

There are many varieties of stretches for any given muscle, depending on which technique you choose. The following are descriptions and illustrations of 10 static stretching exercises that will benefit all the key muscles of the body and improve performance in a wide variety of sports and physical activities. The stretches outlined here are all safe and effective, designed not to stress any of the potentially vulnerable areas of the body, especially the joints.

SHOULDER/UPPER BACK STRETCH

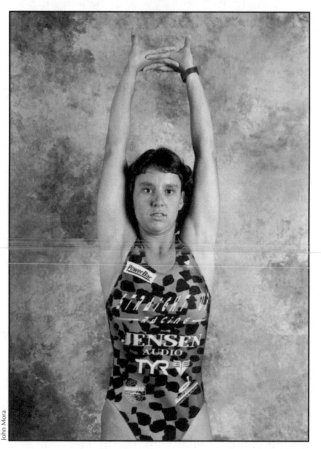

John Mora

Procedure: While standing, clasp your hands behind your neck so that the palms face outward. Straighten your arms and lift upward until you feel a mild pull throughout your upper body. Hold this position for 15-30 s. Then concentrate on pulling your right arm slightly more, hold the position, and repeat the motion with your left arm. As you pull on each arm, you should feel a mild stretch in different areas of your shoulders and upper back.

SHOULDER/CHEST STRETCH

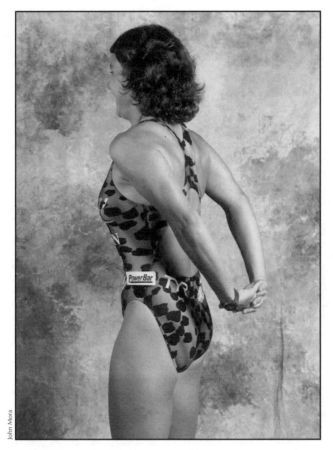

John Mora

Procedure: While standing, clasp your hands behind your back, palms facing upward. Gradually straighten your arms and lift upward and out until you feel a slight discomfort, and hold that position for 15-30 s.

UPPER LEG/HAMSTRING STRETCH

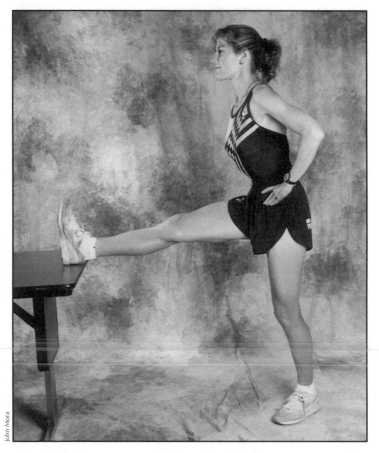

Procedure: Place your leg on a bench or sturdy surface, making sure your foot is not raised higher than waist level. Keep the back leg slightly bent. While maintaining a pelvic tilt, lean into the stretch from your hips. Keep a neutral spine and don't round your back. Be careful not to hyperextend the knee of the stretched leg. Hold for 15-30 s and repeat with the other leg.

QUADRICEPS STRETCH

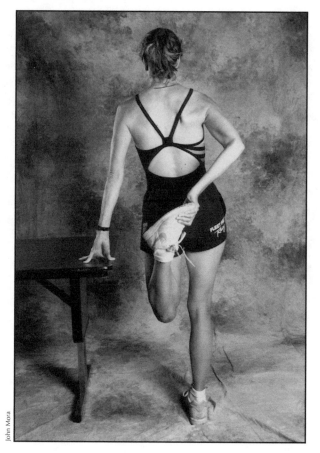

John Mora

Procedure: Stand while holding onto a wall or a tabletop surface. Reach around your body with your right hand and grab your left foot above the ankle. Gently pull your foot close to your buttocks. Make sure both hips are parallel with the floor and that your supporting leg is slightly bent. Hold for 15-30 s and repeat with the other leg.

POSTERIOR SHOULDER/TRAPEZIUS STRETCH

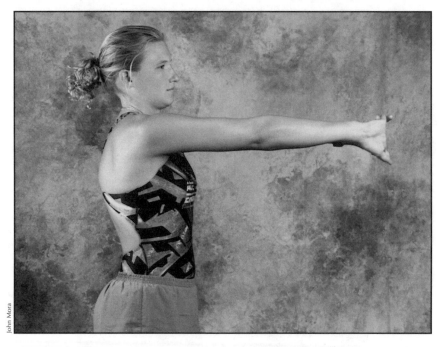

Procedure: While standing, clasp your hands straight forward in front of your body, palms out. Keep your shoulders down and hold to the point of tightness for 15-30 s.

SHOULDER/TRICEPS STRETCH

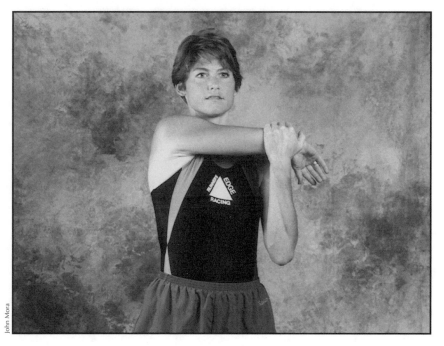

John Mora

Procedure: Place one hand on the opposite arm and gently pull your elbow across your chest and stretch to the opposite shoulder. Hold for 15-30 s and repeat with the other arm.

TRICEPS STRETCH

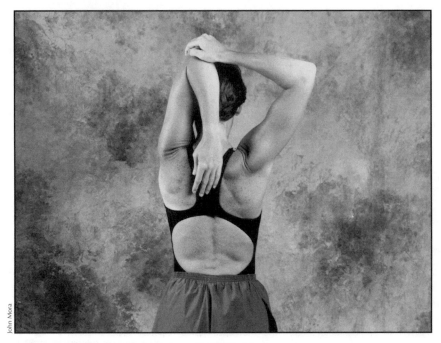

John Mora

Procedure: Holding the elbow of one arm with the opposite hand, point the elbow toward the ceiling and stretch. Hold for 15-30 s and repeat with the other arm.

HIP FLEXOR STRETCH

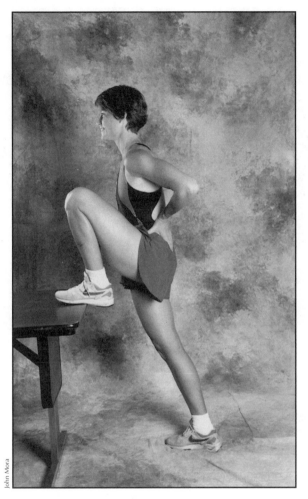

Procedure: In a standing position, place one foot up on a sturdy surface and bend the knee while the supporting leg remains pointed straight ahead. Move the hips forward until you feel the stretch on the hip of the supporting leg. Make sure the hip stays square to the front and doesn't rotate out of the forward plane. Hold for 15-30 s and repeat with the other leg.

GROIN STRETCH

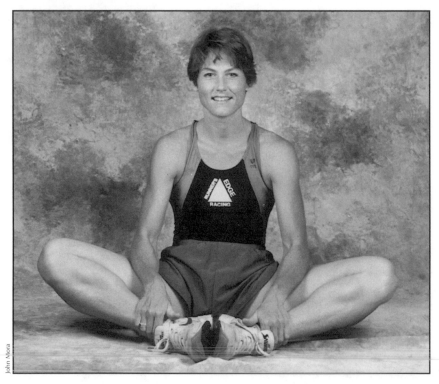

John Mora

Procedure: In a seated position, place the soles of your feet together. Hold them above the ankle while pressing on the inside of the thigh with your elbows for 15-30 s.

BACK/HIP STRETCH

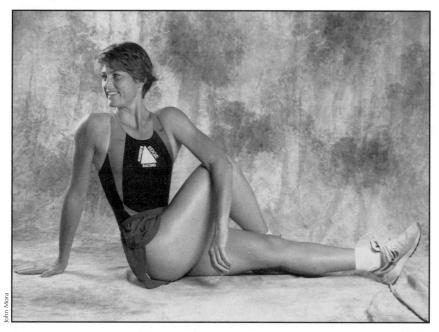

John Mora

Procedure: Start with both legs straight and bend your right leg. Cross your right foot over and rest it next to the outside of your left knee. Place your left elbow on the outside of your upper right thigh, just above the knee. Press into the stretch. Place your right hand behind the hip and turn your head and torso to the point of tightness. Simultaneously rotate your upper body toward your right hand and arm. Lift up out of the rib cage and hold to the point of tightness for 15-30 s. Repeat using the same position with the opposite leg.

PILATES: A FLEXIBILITY ALTERNATIVE

In addition to the static stretching exercises outlined in this chapter, I've recently become involved in a form of exercise that increases flexibility and strength simultaneously. It's called Pilates (pronounced *Pilahtees*), and it was invented by German-born Joseph Pilates.

Pilates was originally developed to aid in the rehabilitation of injured soldiers, but dancers such as Martha Graham, as well as professional athletes, have become attracted to the many strengthening and flexibility benefits of this technique. Joseph Pilates, who came from a sports background, has since refined his system for conditioning the fit body by working with orthopedic specialists in New York.

In recent years, Pilates has become an integral part of training for competitors in a variety of demanding sports: football, skating, volleyball, and triathlon. I was initially drawn to Pilates 2 years ago by Julian Littleford, a former principal dancer with Martha Graham who now runs a Pilates studio, J.L. Body Conditioning in Del Mar, California.

Julian sums up the purpose of this increasingly popular exercise as a way to "strengthen the muscles that are weak, elongate those that are short, and realign and balance your body." In reference to the important benefits to the back muscles with this form of exercise, Joseph Pilates once said, "You are as old as your spine feels. Back pain makes you old fast. If the spine is pliable, you can work out, swim, run, dance and do gardening without fear of aging."

Briefly, here are some of the benefits of Pilates work:

- Increases correct alignment. Repetitive motion can cause irregular muscular development, which is corrected by balancing the body.
- Helps prevent injury.
- Teaches correct breathing technique.
- Simultaneously strengthens muscles while increasing flexibility.
- Integrates the mental aspect of exercise. Teaches harmony between the mind and body.

PILATES PRINCIPLES

The following are the principles upon which the Pilates program is based:

- Pilates is completely nonimpact and non-weight-bearing. It is gentle enough for pregnant women, difficult enough to challenge very fit athletes, and safe enough for athletes in need of rehabilitation from an injury.

- It is based on the principle of variable resistance, so anyone at any age or level of fitness can participate.

- A system of springs and pulleys—rather than weights—is used for resistance. With most weight systems, you must contract the muscle, then let it relax. With Pilates, you have to control the resistance both ways. Because of this, it takes fewer repetitions to see results.

- Pilates is a very energy-efficient exercise. Most activities are done lying down to keep the body in perfect alignment, so there is little wasted energy.

- The nature of this method allows you to identify the muscle groups that need strengthening and stretching. Imbalances show up rapidly, and it is impossible to cheat with the equipment; if you favor one side of your body, it will be immediately obvious.

- Pilates combines the Eastern emphasis on concentration and attention to breathing with the Western approach of working muscles hard to develop a fit body.

- The correct breathing techniques taught in Pilates help flush out lactic acid from the muscles and prevent soreness after a workout.

- Pilates exercises are designed with the entire body in mind. The movements are devised to help the various muscle groups move in natural harmony with other parts of the body. This differs from many exercises that attempt to isolate one muscle group or one section of the body without regard to the body as a whole.

- Pilates works from the inside out, strengthening and balancing the core muscles of the body first, then working out toward other muscle groups.

Unlike other exercise and flexibility programs, Pilates cannot be taught at home; it requires a studio with custom-built equipment and the necessary expansive floor space. Also, a qualified instructor must be present at all times, and a second person is required to recognize when the activities are being performed out of alignment, a key factor with this type of work.

Pilates is an increasingly popular form of exercise, and a studio can most likely be found in your area. Overall, Pilates is a complete exercise, with benefits that affect all three components of the Peak Fitness Triangle. I highly recommend Pilates as a supplement to your peak fitness training. (See the appendix for information on locating a Pilates studio near you.)

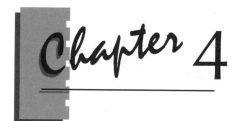

Chapter 4

Strength Training

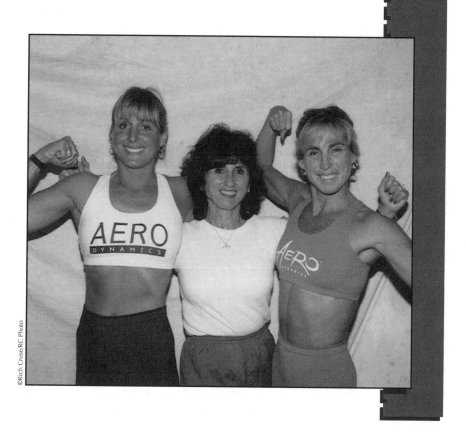

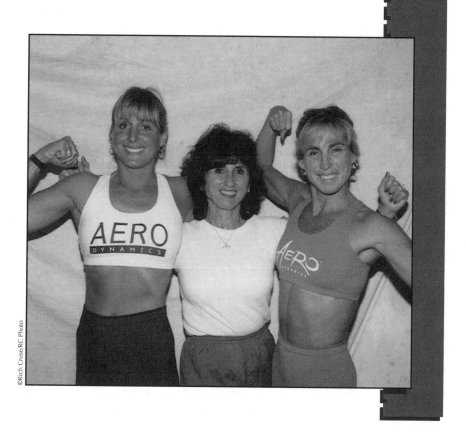

©Rich Cruse/RC Photo

As mentioned in chapter 2, my stress fracture injury was a major factor in my commitment to strength training. I can directly attribute my victory at the Gatorade® Ironman World Championship Triathlon the following fall to my work in the weight room.

My mentor, teacher, and friend, who has guided me through the complicated and technical world of weight training, is Diane Buchta. Diane is a certified fitness specialist and strength training guru from La Jolla, California. She has been teaching and working with weight training to improve her own fitness and the fitness of others for 16 years. Her clients include Mark Allen, Joy Hansen, Paul Huddle, Wolfgang Dittrich, Julia Anne White, and even the famous 91-year-young baby-book author, Dr. Benjamin Spock.

In this chapter, I'll share what Diane has taught me, outlining the benefits, general principles, and tips associated with weight training. Then I'll provide a comprehensive, five-phase weight training program designed by Diane Buchta. (Remember, always consult with your physician before beginning any new exercise program.) Additional information will be supplied on some important abdominal exercises.

Sound technical? Granted, weight training is a fairly technical activity, but don't run for the hills before you give it a try. If strength training has been a low priority in your exercise program, be assured that it can significantly improve your performance.

AFRAID OF BEING MUSCLE-BOUND? FEAR NOT.

A fallacy regarding the strength training component of peak fitness is that it will make you muscle-bound, supposedly leading to loss of coordination and flexibility.

Nothing can be further from the truth. First, coordination is a function of your brain's ability to coordinate your muscles, and no matter how large your muscles get, this vital function will not be impaired.

Second, flexibility is a product of your range of motion. When you are weight training, whether with free weights or a machine such as Nautilus or Universal, you are moving your body through a full range of motion. So, rather than causing inflexibility, strength training increases range of motion, thus increasing flexibility.

With greater flexibility and added strength, you may find that your propensity for injury is greatly decreased. Injury is often the result not only of overburdened muscles but of areas of your body being too tight or too weak, or more than likely, a dangerous combination of both.

THE BENEFITS

When you embark on a strength training program, you'll find that weight training routines can be easily tailored to your individual needs and capacities. And progress usually occurs in a relatively short time. Additionally, you'll experience many psychological benefits to weight training. It can enhance your poise, self-discipline, self-confidence, and self-esteem.

As you can tell, I'm sold on the advantages of partaking in a strength training program. Once you examine the following benefits, I'm sure you will be, too.

HELPS YOU MAINTAIN GOOD HEALTH

Arguably, the greatest benefit of weight training is that it increases your metabolic rate, the rate at which you burn calories. The more lean, strong muscle you build, the higher your metabolism. Your metabolic rate remains higher not just when you exercise but throughout the entire day, even when you sleep.

With the gradual slowdown in metabolism as you age, you can count on a 3% to 5% decrease in the rate of caloric "burnoff" each decade. For every pound of muscle you can add and maintain, you can eat 50 calories more. (How's that for incentive?) However, for every pound of muscle you lose from inactivity or aging, you must decrease your daily calorie intake by 50.

A study published in the *Archives of Internal Medicine* suggests that weight training also may be beneficial in reducing heart disease. Researchers had a group of women ages 28 to 39 work out for an hour on weights, three times a week. After a 5-month period, the LDL cholesterol levels of the women had significantly dropped. (LDL is the "bad" cholesterol that has been linked to heart disease.)

Weight training, when done correctly, can also improve your flexibility by strengthening and moving joints through their full range of motion. This, coupled with the fact that weight training can greatly improve your strength, is particularly helpful to those who are physically underdeveloped.

COUNTERACTS THE EFFECTS OF AGING

Numerous benefits of strength training for older athletes have been well-documented.

Until 1990, the prestigious American College of Sports Medicine (ACSM) prescribed only cardiovascular exercise to combat effects of aging. But after a decade of research, the ACSM revised its guidelines. Instead of recommending only cardiovascular exercise to enhance fitness levels, strength training (as well as flexibility training) has been added to the ACSM guidelines. While cardiovascular exercise contributes to our fitness by elevating metabolism levels for up to 4 hr after exercise, strength training increases our metabolic rate 24 hr a day. So besides improvements in overall health and fitness—not to mention a strong and great-looking body—the addition of strength training can give you a nutritional cushion.

With aging, many people experience a significant decrease in muscle mass. In an interview published in *Weight Watchers Magazine*, Wayne Westcott, PhD, national strength training consultant to the YMCA, stated that women past the age of 30 can lose a half pound of muscle every year if not participating in resistance exercises.

Research at Tufts University, as reported in *Arthritis Today*, concludes that people with certain forms of arthritis can benefit from increasing muscle mass through weight training.

Weight training also may help prevent osteoporosis and contributes to a strong musculoskeletal system, increasing bone density and strengthening the connective tissue surrounding joints. This is especially important to female masters athletes.

IMPROVES PERFORMANCE

A well-chosen sequence of weight exercises done regularly over time can improve your performance in endurance sports. Muscles release energy and originate movement, so strengthening your muscles will make you faster and more powerful.

A recent study at the University of Maryland demonstrated that cyclists improved their performances with the addition of a weight training program. Strength training elevated their anaerobic threshold by 12%, enabling them to go longer on a bicycle ergometer.

GUARDS AGAINST INJURY

A strong muscular system provides protection against injury, no matter what your sport. Doing any activity often enough or long enough causes wear and tear on the muscles and joints involved.

For example, long-distance running stresses the rear leg muscles and deemphasizes front leg muscles. The continuous muscle imbalance decreases knee joint stability and increases the risk of injury. A strength training exercise such as leg extensions can help strengthen the typically weak knee joint of a long-distance runner. By working the quadriceps and other muscles that surround the kneecap, the area is stabilized and correct tracking is more likely.

DESIGNING YOUR PROGRAM

Before adding any new exercise activity to your regular routine, it's necessary to go over some ground rules. Ideally, you should stick to the program presented here, but at the very least, maintain some kind of strength training schedule. If you let it slide, your muscles will become deconditioned after 6 to 8 weeks.

Remember, weight training should not be your only exercise activity if you want to achieve peak fitness. It should be one of the three components of peak fitness, in addition to flexibility training and cardiovascular exercise.

Before diving into the mechanics of the strength training program, let's look at some general principles and guidelines to keep in mind when designing your weight training program.

SAFETY FIRST

Safety should be your first concern. Fortunately, the "no pain, no gain" era in exercise is a thing of the past. If it hurts too much, don't do it, or ask a qualified instructor to help you or show you an alternative exercise. Likewise, choose a weight that is a challenge, not a strain.

Do not perform more than 10 exercises in the beginning of your program. The ACSM recommends one set of 8 to 12 repetitions of 8 to 10 different exercises at least twice a week as a minimum.

A good warm-up and cooldown are important. Spend some time stretching before and after your strength training workout. Refer to the stretching exercises in chapter 3. Also, if you are at a health club or gym and find yourself waiting for a machine or barbell, don't let your muscles cool down. Use a form of "active rest" and stretch during these delays.

PRACTICE PROPER TECHNIQUE

Begin working on the large muscle groups and then progress to the middle and small muscle groups. For example, a workout progression might go like this: quadriceps, hamstrings, chest, biceps, then wrists. There are two main reasons for this: (a) the larger muscle groups will provide the greatest strength gains and produce greater increases in metabolic rate and, therefore, should be worked on first; and (b) susceptibility to injury is greatly decreased if the larger muscle groups are worked on first.

Be patient and progress gradually at a reasonable pace. It's better to get from point A to point B safely and slowly than to injure yourself because you tried to get there too fast. When you injure yourself due to haste, you increase the time it takes to get where you wanted to go anyway, thus defeating your original purpose.

Increase poundage and repetitions slowly. Soreness and stiffness need not occur as long as you ease into the program. Your increases in poundage and/or repetitions should be incremental but gradual. Increases should also reflect the goals of your program. When increasing repetitions, expect to decrease poundage at first, then gradually increase weights 5% to 10% for upper body exercise and 10% to 20% for lower body exercises.

Always work the muscles through the full range of motion. Form is more important than the amount of weight. If you sacrifice your form to lift a heavier weight, you are cheating yourself out of the full benefit of strength training and you increase the risk of injuring yourself.

The execution of each exercise and the speed of the movement should be slow and controlled. Use the 2/4 rule: count out 2 s in the first phase of lifting (or pushing, pulling) and 4 s to complete the exercise when lowering (or pulling, pushing).

Use correct breathing technique. Exhale at the point of effort, when the weight is being lifted (pushed, pulled) against gravity. Inhale while you lower (pull, push) the weight.

GET ENOUGH REST

It is important to rest between sets. Resting for 30 s to 1 min is fine, depending on the phase in which you are working. If you are performing a particularly intense workout, a 2- to 4-min rest between sets may be needed. Another way of resting major muscle groups is to alternate between upper body and lower body exercises. A third option is to alternate between agonistic and antagonistic muscles (for example, biceps to triceps or quadriceps to hamstrings).

Get enough rest between workouts, too. Take at least 48 hr but no more than 72 hr to recover. Although I'll go into the importance of rest in greater detail in chapter 7, I want to stress here that rest is the most significant ingredient in training your muscles with weights. It is actually during rest, not during your workout, that your body absorbs the training and becomes stronger.

VARY YOUR EQUIPMENT

Use a variety of equipment. Visit any health club and you'll soon see that there is a wide selection of exercise machines. Don't let that intimidate you. Rather, set about finding the machines or free weight equipment that you feel most comfortable working on. Consider factors that affect comfort such as the handles, padding, method of resistance, and machine design.

There is an ongoing debate in the weight training world about whether free weights or machines are better. Although the debate may never end, the truth is that both are good, but both have limitations.

The advantage of free weights is that you use peripheral muscles that help with balance, coordination, and agility. Machines have fixed movement planes that do not allow the muscles to coordinate and develop in the same way that free weights do. The disadvantages of free weights are that they make it harder for the novice to learn correct form and there is greater risk of injury because there is no fixed axis of rotation.

THE PEAK FITNESS PROGRAM

This weight training program was designed and modified by my strength training coach, Diane Buchta. It is based on the principle of *periodization*, which means a division of training into smaller, more manageable segments or phases. Periodization also implies that you define and dedicate each phase to a specific training goal.

It's essential for you to understand that, by its very nature, a weight training program based on periodization requires a long-term commitment. It is based on phases that target a specific goal, leading to long-term performance improvements in your cardiovascular sport.

Don't be frightened or intimidated by the technical nature of weight training represented in the sample log pages and workout schedules presented here and in chapter 8. After you've become familiar with the program, you will enjoy using these practical and easy-to-understand tools.

THE PEAK FITNESS STRENGTH TRAINING LOG

Keeping a log is important to success in weight training. It's an essential tool for tracking and measuring your progress. There are five phases in the Peak Fitness Training Program described in the next section. In each description, you'll find a sample log page. You can duplicate it or use it as a guide to creating your own weight training log.

Sample Log Page	Week 1		1 set 12 reps	Week 2		2 sets 12 reps
	Date *1/3*	*1/5*	*1/7*	*1/10*	*1/12*	*1/14*
Lat Pulldown	Weight *50*	*50*	*50*	*50*	*60*	*60*
Leg Extension	*60*	*60*	*65*	*65*	*70*	*70*
Bench Press	*70*	*70*	*70*	*75*	*75*	*75*

Make sure to keep track of your workouts and the pounds you lift in your log pages. By filling in your training log at the end of each session, you can measure your progress at each phase.

Reprinted with permission of Kevin Wendle productions.

STRENGTH TRAINING EXERCISES

The following exercises, listed from large to small muscle groups, are the core weight training exercises you will perform throughout most phases of the program. These exercises will improve muscular strength and endurance in almost any sport. In later phases, additional exercises will be recommended. Refer to the training log in each phase and perform only the exercises that are listed.

When an *(alt)* is designated, you have the option of performing the alternative exercise, which may include the use of free weights.

In the first phase, the acclimation phase, the primary goal is to accustom the body to resistance training. Exercises marked with an asterisk (*) should not be performed until the beginning of Week 3 of the program.

LARGE MUSCLE GROUPS

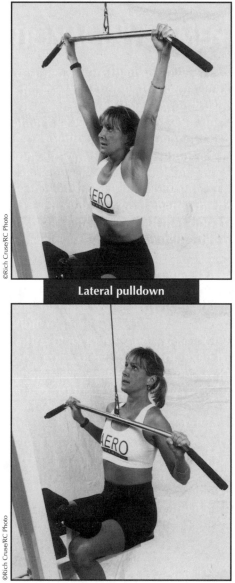

Lateral pulldown

©Rich Cruse/RC Photo

©Rich Cruse/RC Photo

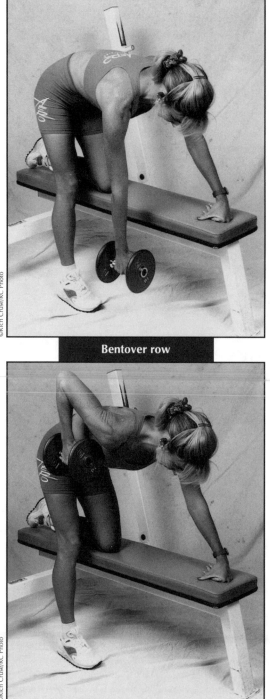

Bentover row

©Rich Cruse/RC Photo

©Rich Cruse/RC Photo

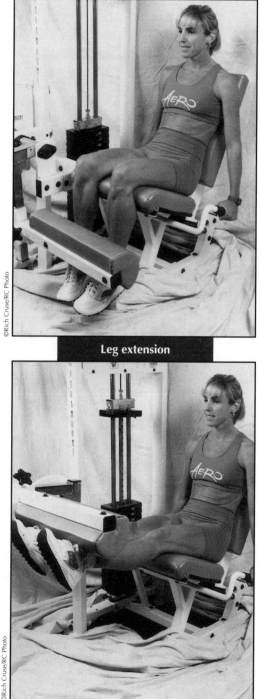

©Rich Cruse/RC Photo

Leg extension

©Rich Cruse/RC Photo

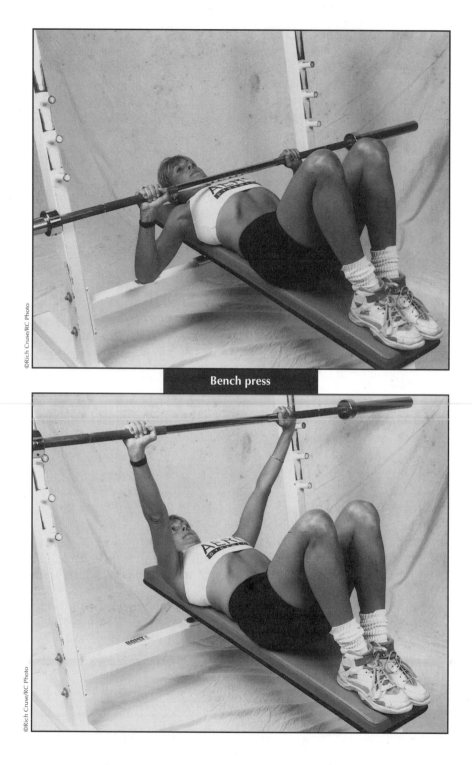

Bench press

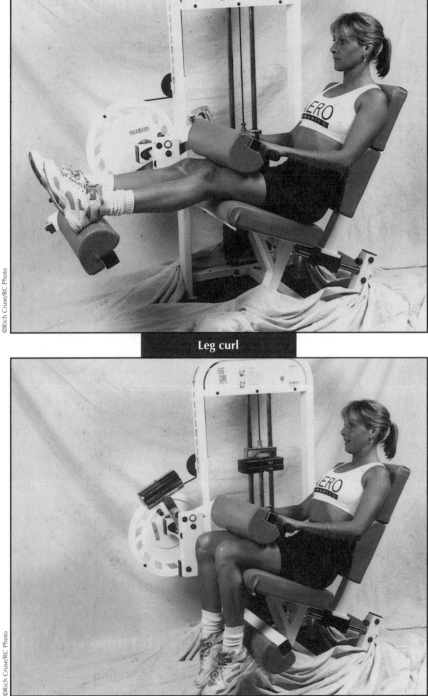

©Rich Cruse/RC Photo

©Rich Cruse/RC Photo

Leg curl

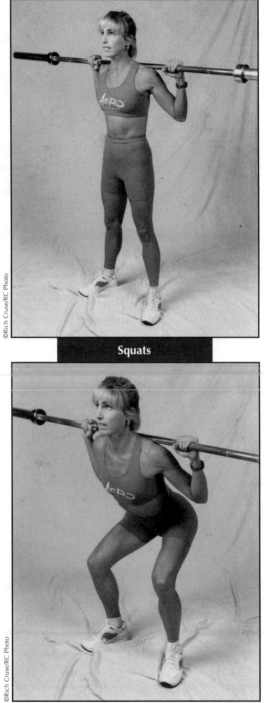

©Rich Cruse/RC Photo

Squats

©Rich Cruse/RC Photo

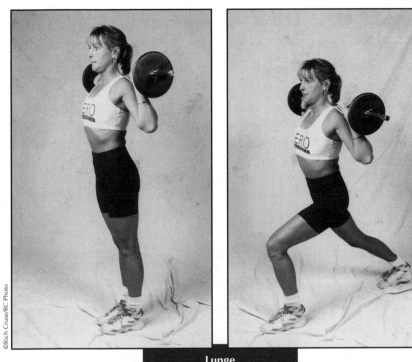

Lunge

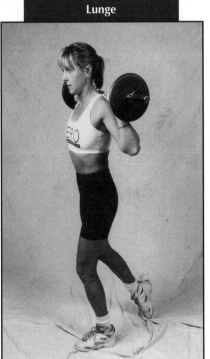

MIDDLE MUSCLE GROUPS

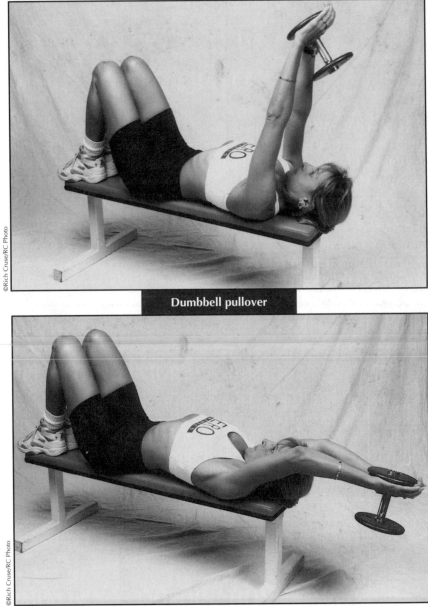

Dumbbell pullover

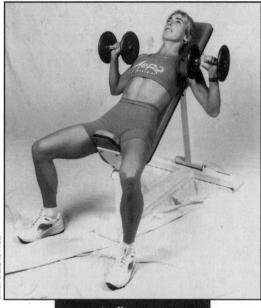

Incline press

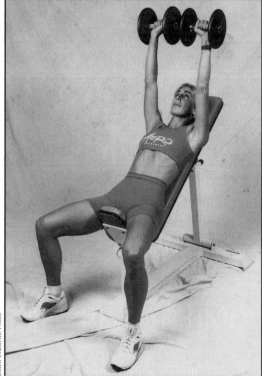

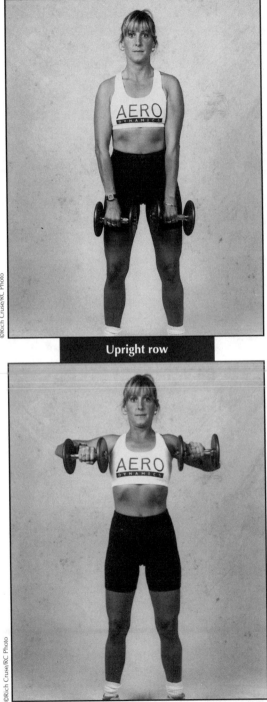

©Rich Cruse/RC Photo

Upright row

©Rich Cruse/RC Photo

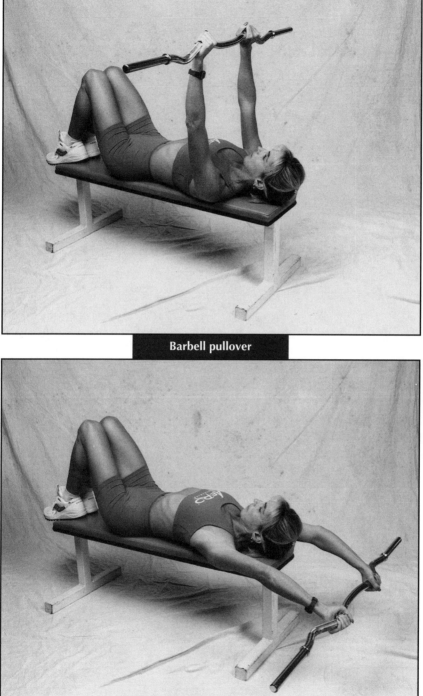

©Rich Cruse/RC Photo

Barbell pullover

©Rich Cruse/RC Photo

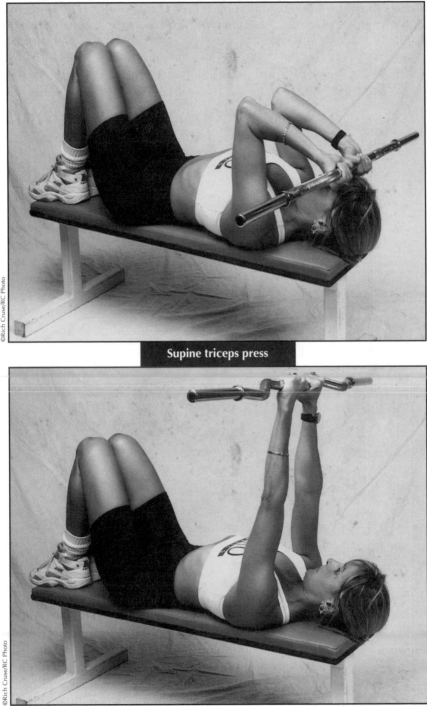

Supine triceps press

©Rich Cruse/RC Photo

©Rich Cruse/RC Photo

SMALL MUSCLE GROUPS

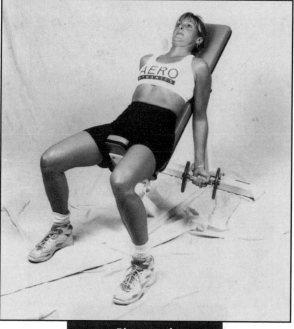

©Rich Cruse/RC Photo

Biceps curl

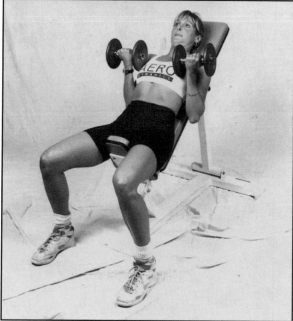

©Rich Cruse/RC Photo

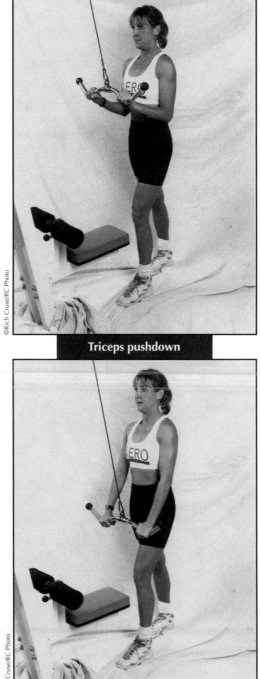

Triceps pushdown

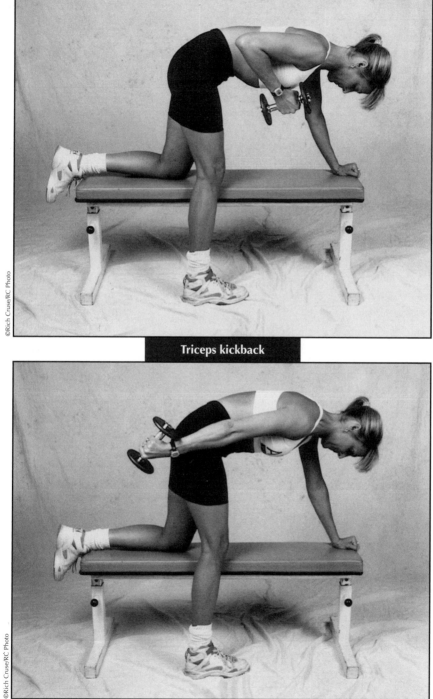

©Rich Cruse/RC Photo

Triceps kickback

©Rich Cruse/RC Photo

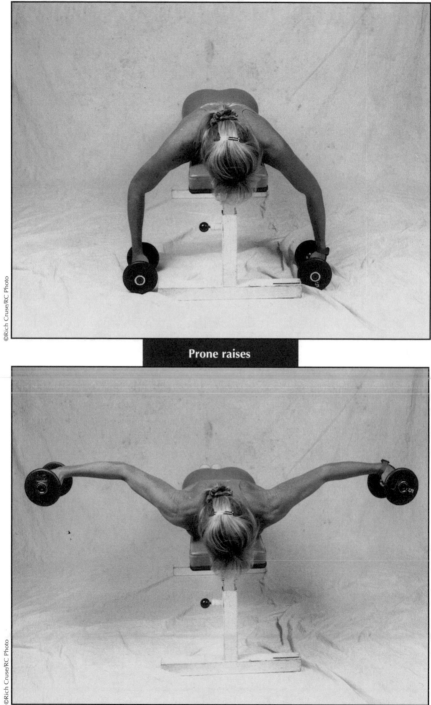

Prone raises

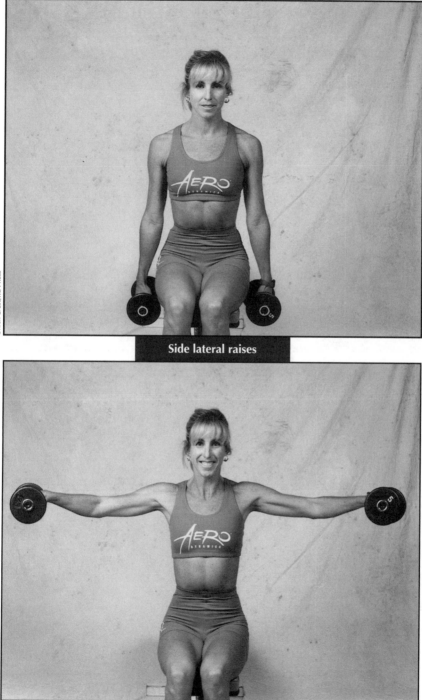

Side lateral raises

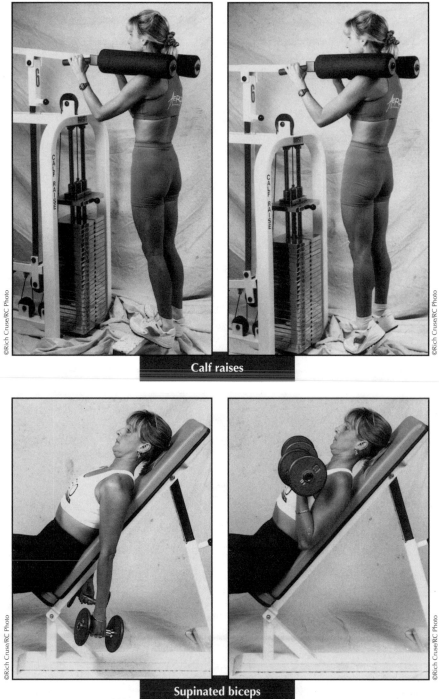

Calf raises

Supinated biceps

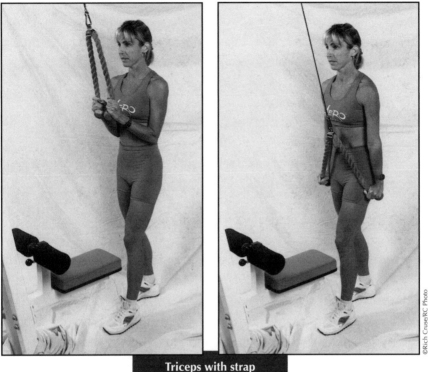

©Rich Cruse/RC Photo

©Rich Cruse/RC Photo

Triceps with strap

PHASE 1: ACCLIMATION `Pages 98-99`

Purpose: To accustom the neuromuscular system to the demands of the latter stages; to learn the skills and techniques of resistance training; to establish a strength training base.

Duration: 5 weeks

Frequency: The most dramatic improvements will occur if you schedule three weight sessions a week. Schedule them for every other day to allow for the necessary recovery time. Good results will still occur if you work out twice a week.

Workout Structure: Perform the following workout every other day:

- Week 1: One set of 12 repetitions (reps).
- Week 2: Two sets of 12 reps.
- Weeks 3 through 5: Three sets of 12 reps.

Things to Remember:

- Begin every workout with a warm-up consisting of at least 5 to 10 min of aerobic exercise followed by stretching. Never start a weight training workout cold.
- Gradually increase the weight after you've reached three sets of 12 repetitions in Week 3.
- Schedule your weight training for the time of day when you have the most energy.
- If you're training at a health club, schedule your workout for a time of day when it is least likely to be crowded.

PHASE 2: STRENGTH AND ENDURANCE   Pages 100-101

Purpose: The focus of this phase is to enhance your endurance by working on "slow-twitch" muscle fibers.

Duration: 4 to 5 weeks

Frequency: If you've been working out with weights twice a week, consider increasing the frequency to three times a week.

Workout Structure: Think "speed" between exercises (not during the actual motion). Finish your reps and go on to the next exercise.

- Week 6: Two sets of 15 reps.
- Weeks 7 through 10: Two to three sets of 20 reps.
- Perform one to three sets of 20 reps of abdominals. For press-ups, do two sets of 10 reps. (Abdominals and press-ups are discussed later in this chapter.)

Things to Remember:

- You will be increasing the number of repetitions per set in this phase, so you can expect to decrease the number of pounds you lift at first.
- Continue to increase the weight gradually but be careful not to overreact to improvements in strength and make increases that are too dramatic.
- Your level of discomfort when lifting weights should be moderate to light. Choose a weight that works your muscles to fatigue. If it hurts too much, you're probably lifting too much weight.

- Everyone has good days and bad days. Most often this is affected by mood or other mental variables. The important thing is to stick with your program, no matter what your mood.

PHASE 3: POWER AND ENDURANCE Pages 102-103

Purpose: To increase muscle hypertrophy. (If physical demands are placed upon a muscle often enough, physiological changes occur that can result in an increase in size. That increase is called muscle hypertrophy.) A second purpose is to establish strength and power at peak levels.

Duration: 4 to 6 weeks

Frequency: Increase to (or maintain) a frequency of three times a week.

Workout Structure: In this phase, you will be decreasing the repetitions but increasing the intensity or poundage. "Powered" sets are those in which the weight is increased substantially, so expect to add about 30% more weight to each exercise. Refer to the training log and power only those specific exercises targeted for that day.

The other exercises are designed for endurance, so execute two sets of 20 repetitions. If you work out a third day, you should just do 2×20, thinking "speed" between sets. Do not power train three days a week.

Use the following workout structure for designated powered exercises:

- Week 11: Two sets of 6 reps.
- Week 12: Three sets of 6 reps.
- Weeks 13 through 15: Three sets of 8 reps.
- For exercises during a workout that are not powered, perform two sets of 20 repetitions.

Things to Remember:

- Extended recovery time may be necessary between powered exercises. A 2- to 4-min recovery is appropriate. Don't alternate from upper to lower or agonist to antagonist in the powered exercises but do so for the 2×20 endurance sets.
- On exercises that are being powered, execute to the point of muscle failure but keep proper form. You want the ultimate challenge to the muscle while maintaining correct technique.

- Naturally, your level of discomfort in this phase will be higher, but if you experience intense pain, chances are you've increased the weight too rapidly.

- Women are generally afraid of "bulking up," so this phase may be less appealing to some. You will notice significant muscle size increases—a necessary side effect of this type of training. In most instances, the bulk is "chiseled away" later with cardiovascular conditioning and in the following peak power phase, while still allowing you to maintain greater muscular strength and power.

- In this phase, you may need to use a spotter when training on free weights.

"HERE SPOT"

A necessary aspect of free weight training is the use of a spotter. A good spotter is someone who will protect you as well as motivate you to lift just one more rep when your arms feel like burning matchsticks.

If you don't have a weight training partner, the best way to find a spotter is to look for someone who is alone in the free weight training area of your health club. Chances are, he or she will be looking for a spotter as well. If you're married and work out at home, get your spouse or adult son or daughter involved.

Some tips on spotting:

- Make sure your spotter can handle the weight you are using and that he or she understands proper technique.

- Spotters should never stand on the equipment. They should always be in a correct position to help you, if needed.

- A spotter may not have to do anything during most workout sessions. But, because at any moment a situation could arise where you do need your partner's help, make sure your spotter doesn't get careless. A spotter should always be in a ready stance when you are lifting. Of course, the same goes for you when you are spotting.

PHASE 4: PEAK POWER | *Pages 104-105* |

Purpose: To maintain your gains in strength and power. The focus is on upper body exercises. This will allow you to concentrate on intense cardiovascular training in sports that involve the lower body.

Duration: 5 weeks

Frequency: Cut down on the frequency in this stage to allow for recovery and avoid burnout. Workouts should be done twice a week, with rest periods of 3 to 4 days.

Workout Structure: With the exception of lunges, drop all lower body weight training exercises you have been doing so far and limit your total number of exercises to 10. As in the strength and endurance phase, speed is a critical factor, so cut down on the duration of your rest interval between reps. Also, while still using caution and control, take 2 s to lift and 2 s to lower the weight.

- Weeks 16 through 20: Two sets of 12 reps.
- For abdominal exercises, perform two to four sets of 20 repetitions. Do 10 reps of press-ups.

Things to Remember:

- This phase should be scheduled in your yearly plan to correspond with interval or high-intensity workouts in your cardiovascular activities.
- If you are a runner, a cyclist, a triathlete, or a participant in any sport that depends primarily on the lower body, your interval and high-intensity cardiovascular workout will take a toll on your legs. With the exception of lunges, do not perform any lower body weight training exercises. Lunges will help you maintain your lower body strength and still allow your legs the time they need to recover from your hard cardiovascular workout.

PHASE 5: MAINTENANCE | *Pages 104-105* |

Purpose: To maintain strength, endurance, and power gained from the previous phases throughout your endurance racing season.

Duration: 5 weeks (for racers it may require more time, depending on the length of your season)

Frequency: Maintain strength by consistently working out with weights every 4 to 5 days.

Workout Structure: For each week of this phase, perform one set of 12 reps each of the exercises listed in the acclimation phase training log. If pressed for time, do only the six exercises marked with a (Δ), which are the most essential. If time permits, perform the entire workout.

Things to Remember:

- The key to maintaining the gains from previous phases is to listen to your body. Don't push too hard if you feel pain or let yourself get lazy if you feel your strength level declining.

ABDOMINALS: STRENGTHENING THE CORE

Before I knew what a triathlon was, I began taking aerobics classes that integrated an abdominal routine. The hardest thing for everyone in the class was surviving those hellish exercises, which the instructor adapted from a Jane Fonda video. Ever the competitor, I wanted to cruise through them better than anyone else. So I set about working at it, and before long, I was breezing through abdominal exercises while the rest griped and groaned. That routine is still part of my exercise routine. I use the Fonda workout religiously and do my abdominal exercises three times a week after every run. This habit has helped me significantly throughout my career.

The abdominal muscles, or "abs," are the core or center of body strength. They are referred to as the rectis abdominis and the internal and external oblique muscles (see p. 91). Think of the rectus abdominis as a long, flat sheet of muscle that extends from your breastbone to your hipbone and has an upper and lower region. The side regions are the external and internal obliques. A weakness in this core area will limit the efficiency of all other working muscles.

If you were to ask most people "What about your body would you most like to change?" the answer would probably be their abdominal region. There is a proliferation of quick-fix plans, gadgets, and programs designed to reduce the size of abs, but most of these "miracle" products are based on the incorrect assumption that you can easily isolate this section of the body. These kinds of products and programs lead to frustration caused by unrealistic expectations.

That's not to say that the situation is hopeless—far from it. If you want to improve the appearance of your abs and strengthen your core, you need to take a different, more holistic approach. Researchers Douglas

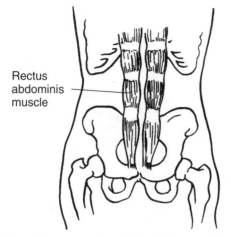

Rectus
abdominis
muscle

Exercising your rectus abdominis is one of the keys
to strengthening your "core," which is beneficial to
virtually every form of exercise.

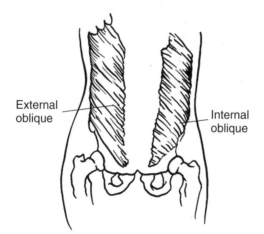

External
oblique

Internal
oblique

Many popular exercises neglect the vital side regions
of the abdominal area. The forthcoming exercises are
designed to strengthen the entire abdominal region,
including the external and internal obliques.

Brooks, MS, and Candice Copeland-Brooks advocate the need to focus
on the trunk region as a whole rather than on just the abdominals.

More specifically, this means strengthening both the anterior
(abdominals) and posterior musculature of the abdominal section, an
approach known as trunk stabilization. The approach takes into
account that the whole abdominal group is important in achieving
proper spinal alignment and pelvic stability in the trunk.

Setup: Lie on the floor and tilt your pelvis so that your back is comfortable and in a neutral position. Place a rolled-up towel under your spine if you experience any discomfort. Next, contract your abdominals. Remember to stabilize the pelvic or core area when doing all abdominal work.

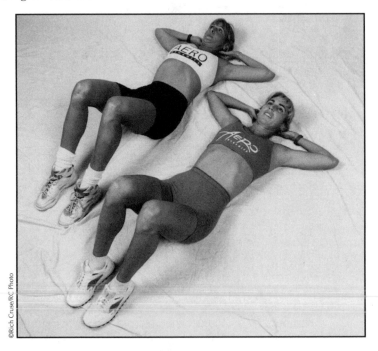

Workout Structure: Include at least three sessions a week of abdominal exercises—more, if possible. Unless indicated otherwise in previous phases, start with one set of 20 repetitions of each abdominal exercise shown here. Gradually work your way up to three or four sets of 20 reps of each exercise.

Things to Remember:

- Pay attention to the order in which you work the muscles. Work the abdominals starting with the lower portion, then the middle, and finally the upper abs. The muscle fibers of the upper abdominal region are involved in all abdominal exercises and are the easiest to train. This is why it's essential to progress in this way—if you start with the upper abs first, you'll be too fatigued to work the lower and middle areas.

- Always follow your ab routine with press-ups to stretch the abdominals and strengthen the back.

Lower abdominal region: Keep your head stable and your trunk controlled and bend both legs until your feet are flat on the floor a few inches from your buttocks. Bring one leg up toward your chest, then lower it back to the floor. Continue alternating legs while contracting the core area. If this is not a challenge, try lifting both legs simultaneously, then lower them as close to the floor as possible.

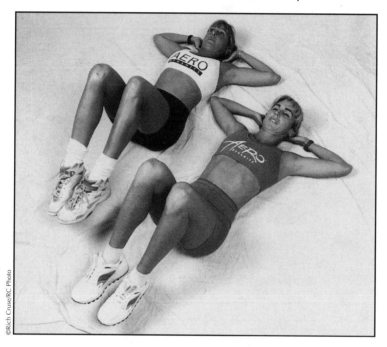

©Rich Cruse/RC Photo

Middle abdominal region (obliques): Place your feet flat on the floor. Bend your knees, keep your back neutral, and contract your abdominals. Place your hands behind your head, elbows open wide, but never pull on your neck. Lift your head, neck, and shoulders off the floor as a single unit. Exhale up and rotate, pointing one shoulder (not your elbow) to the opposite knee. Inhale down and exhale and rotate up to the opposite side.

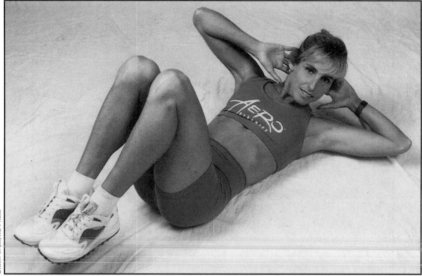

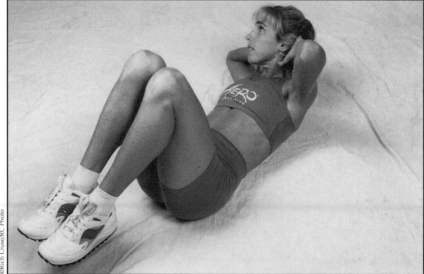

Upper abdominal region: Use the same foot and arm position as in the previous exercise. Look up at the ceiling and visualize an orange under your chin. Exhale up and try to clear your shoulder blades off the floor. Pause and slowly inhale down. Do not jut out your chin.

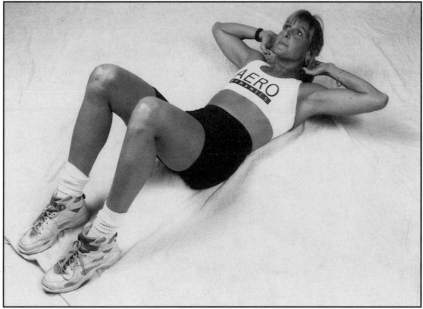

PRESS-UPS: BALANCING YOUR WORKOUT

Press-ups will help you strengthen your back muscles and stretch your abdominals. This is important, considering the essential role back and abdominal muscles play in every form of exercise as well as in everyday activities.

Procedure: *Lie on your stomach with your palms flat. Place your hands under your shoulders and press upward while keeping your pelvis on the mat. Slowly exhale up and inhale down. If you experience pain, stop.*

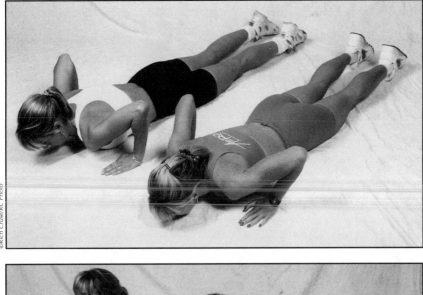

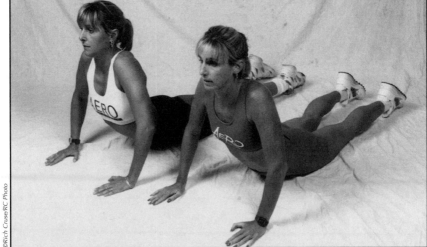

A CONVENIENT WORKOUT
FOR THE TRAVELING ATHLETE

A simple piece of surgical tubing can be a safe, easy, and convenient way to get a great strength workout. I never travel anywhere without my tubing; it serves as a stand-in when I can't get to a gym to do my regular weight workout. Although a piece of tubing that you can get at any medical supply store will work, I recommend spending a few dollars more on tubing specifically designed for this purpose. Tubing is available with handles and door brackets for added safety and comfort, as well as accompanying literature on the various exercises.

Surgical tubing gives you complete access to strength training, either at home or when traveling. It is a convenient way of maintaining and improving strength. Used properly, surgical tubing can train the muscles through an athletic and functional range of motion that helps increase flexibility.

Resistance is increased or decreased by the distance or tension in the tubing when you begin the exercise. The further your distance from the point of attachment or anchor, the more difficult the exercise becomes. You can also increase the resistance by shortening the tubing.

To find out where to purchase surgical tubing with handles, including a brochure of strength training exercises, check the appendix at the back of the book.

ACCLIMATION

		Week 1	1 set 12 reps	Week 2		2 sets 12 reps
		Date				
	Warm-up/Stretch					
Large	Lat pulldown Alt: Bent over row	Weight				
Large	Leg extension*					
Large	Bench press Alt: Dumbbell press					
Large	Leg curl*					
Large	Squats	Begin 3rd week				
Middle	Dumbbell pullover					
Middle	Incline dumbbell press					
Middle	Upright row	Begin 3rd week				
Small	Biceps curl					
Small	Tricep pushdown Alt: Tricep kickback					
Small	Prone raises					
Small	Side lateral raises	Begin 3rd week				
Small	Calf raises	Begin 3rd week				
	Abdominals					
	Press-ups					
	Stretch					

Reprinted with permission of Kevin Wendle production.

PHASE ①

WEEKS 1-5

Week 3		3 sets 12 reps	Week 4		3 sets 12 reps	Week 5		3 sets 12 reps

STRENGTH/ENDURANCE

Follow weekly number of sets **except** as noted for Abs and Press-ups.	Week 6	2 set 15 reps	Week 7	2 sets 20 reps			
	Date						
Warm-up/Stretch							
Lat pulldown	Weight						
Leg extension							
Bench press							
Leg curl							
Squats							
Dumbbell pullover							
Supine tricep press							
Incline press							
Upright row							
Bicep curl							
Supinated bicep							
Tricep pushdown							
Prone raises							
Side lateral raises							
Calf raises							
Abdominals 1-3 sets 20 reps							
Press-ups 2 sets 10 reps							
Stretch							

Large / Middle / Small

PHASE ②

WEEKS 6-10

Week 8		3 sets 20 reps	Week 9		3 sets 20 reps	Week 10		3 sets 20 reps

POWER/ENDURANCE

Perform 2 sets of 20 reps when an exercise for a day is shaded	Week 11		2 sets 6 reps	Week 12		3 sets 6 reps
	Date					
Warm-up/Stretch						
Large — Lat pulldown	Weight					
Leg extension						
Bench press						
Leg curl						
Squats						
Middle — Dumbbell pullover						
Incline dumbbell press						
Upright row						
Small — Biceps curl						
Tricep pushdown						
Tricep with strap						
Prone raises						
Side lateral raises						
Calf raises						
Abdominals						
Press-up						
Stretch						

PHASE ③

WEEKS 11-15

Week 13		3 sets 8 reps	Week 14		3 sets 8 reps	Week 15		3 sets 8 reps

PEAK POWER

Adjust sets and reps as noted for abs and press-ups.	Week 16	2 sets 12 reps	Week 17	2 sets 12 reps
	Date			
Warm-up/Stretch				
Lat pulldown	Weight			
Lunge				
Bench press				
Barbell pullover				
Supine tricep press				
Tricep with strap				
Supinated bicep				
Abdominals (20 reps)				
Press-ups (10 reps)				

• Reduce exercises to 10, but keep intensity high.

MAINTENANCE

		Week 21	1 sets 12 reps	Week 22	1 sets 12 reps
		Date			
	Warm-up/Stretch				
Δ	Lat pulldown	Weight			
	Lunge				
Δ	Bench press				
Δ	Barbell pullover				
Δ	Supine tricep press				
	Tricep with strap				
Δ	Supinated bicep				
Δ	Abdominals (20 reps)				
	Press-ups (10 reps)				

• If pressed for time, do the six basic exercises (Δ).

PHASE ④

WEEKS 16-20

Week 18	2 sets 12 reps	Week 19	2 sets 12 reps	Week 20	2 sets 12 reps

• Do 2 sets of 12 reps for each exercise once every 3-4 days.

PHASE ⑤

WEEKS 21-25

Week 23	1 sets 12 reps	Week 24	1 sets 12 reps	Week 25	1 sets 12 reps

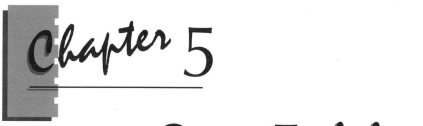

Chapter 5

Cross-Training

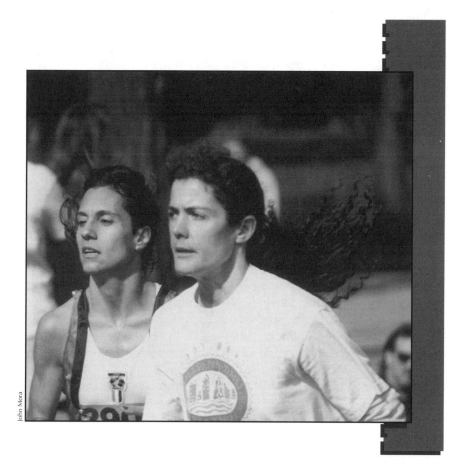

John Mora

Are you a runner who doesn't particularly care for swimming in open water among our aquatic friends—or for that matter, doesn't care for swimming at all? Are you a cyclist who cringes at the very sight of running shoes? Although cross-training is typically associated with triathletes, it's a myth that cross-training should only include swimming, cycling, and running.

As a professional triathlete, my main cardiovascular activities are swimming, biking, and running. I also walk, in-line skate, do aerobics, and mountain bike. Why would I jeopardize my professional career by participating in these other sports? Because they're fun. And besides, participating in these sports during the off-season and a limited amount during the racing season gives me a mental edge over everyone else who's been stroking, pedaling, and pounding too long.

What can cross-training do for you? How can participation in one physical activity help you in another? How can cross-training help you achieve peak fitness?

Whether you're a triathlete shooting for optimum performance or a runner, cyclist, in-line skater, or fitness enthusiast looking for a high level of conditioning, cross-training *can* help you achieve peak fitness.

WHAT IS CROSS-TRAINING?

Although cross-training may seem like a new concept, the history of cross-training goes back to the turn of the century. It was then that physiologists demonstrated the relationship between corresponding muscle groups. Experiments showed that a stationary muscle, such as an arm muscle held in a cast, would show less deterioration when the other healthy arm was exercised at high intensity.

How can this be? There is a spillover effect from the active nerves of healthy muscles that are being exercised intensely to the nerves of the immobile or unhealthy muscles. This spillover stimulation between muscle nerves aids in the recovery of the unhealthy muscles.

Although this phenomenon is not direct proof of the validity of cross-training, the implication is that the body is a total working system, tied together by nerves, muscles, and neuromuscular impulses in ways we still don't understand. This physiological phenomenon lends credence to what triathletes have proven on lakes, roadways, and running trails throughout the world: a structured fitness program that integrates cross-training in a balanced and efficient way can help you achieve a high level of fitness.

Let's look at the physiological facts that reveal how cross-training works. They might provide insight as to the aim of any cross-training program as well as some clues about how to get there. If scientific jargon bores you, or if you run away screaming every time you read a word that ends with -*ology* (hellish visions of your overdisciplining high school biology teacher seared on your mind), try to bear with me. Look at these facts as a general roadmap to peak fitness.

Lesson 1: You remember from biology that muscles can only be relaxed or contracted. Like a light switch, muscles are either on or off.

Lesson 2: Bodily movement comes from two sets of muscles working against each other. One muscle pulls (contracts), initiating movement, while the other muscle opposes the pull (relaxes), eventually pulling the initiating muscle back to its original position.

Lesson 3: To distinguish between the two opposing muscles, let's call the pulling or contracting muscle the agonist muscle and the opposing muscle the antagonist muscle.

Lesson 4: Now let's determine what happens with agonist and antagonist muscles during exercise, using the pedaling motion in cycling as an example. During pedaling, the quadriceps initiate motion, contracting and acting as the agonists. At the same time, the hamstrings in the back of your thighs act as the antagonists.

What do you think will happen to those muscles over time? When you look at the legs of champion cyclists, the first thing you notice is their massive quadriceps, and if you were to test their hamstrings, chances are they would be relatively weak compared to their quads.

Which brings us to the point of lesson 4: agonist muscles are usually much stronger than their antagonist counterparts, creating a substantial muscle imbalance.

Lesson 5: To maximize performance and reach peak fitness, a cross-training regimen must be designed to strengthen both the agonist and antagonist muscles in the right proportions for optimum balance and muscular fitness.

The primary message behind this anatomy lesson: Your body is a complex system that is tied together in many incomprehensible ways. Just as a physician can't look at an injury and make an accurate diagnosis without looking at the entire body, neither can you afford to be narrow-minded about your training.

Cross-training is a dynamic approach to fitness that—because of its balanced approach—is the foundation of peak fitness.

THE BENEFITS

When I entered the sport of triathlon, the variety of workouts helped me get over an aversion I had to pool swimming (for the most part). Some negative high school swim team experiences taught me that the most important benefit of cross-training is the mental variety and balance it gives you. Cross-training can also give you some very tangible and performance-enhancing physical benefits.

FRESH MUSCLES

Every endurance athlete has fallen prey to the effects of prolonged exercise on tired muscles. They often show up as a burning sensation, for example, when your quadriceps feel like they're on fire while cycling up a steep hill. Perhaps you feel it most during an intense interval workout on the running track.

What you're feeling is the result of lactic acid buildup, a natural by-product of strenuous exercise. After periods of prolonged, intense exercise, lactic acid and other metabolic waste products accumulate in tired muscles. Besides causing that burning sensation, this buildup inhibits muscular contraction, which limits your ability to exercise. The result is decreased performance.

Cross-training can help transfer the strain to another muscle group, enlisting fresh muscles to bear the brunt of exercising your body. The result can be exhilarating.

Every competitive triathlete knows the feeling of fatigue that comes toward the end of the swim leg of a race. The last quarter of a swim is especially tiring if you haven't had the luxury of drafting behind another swimmer. Your stroke starts to deteriorate, the waves hit you in the face, and pretty soon you feel as though you're just slapping water and going nowhere.

But once the swim is finished and the race to the transition area begins, there's a rush of available energy. Admittedly, much of this newfound storehouse of power can be attributed to the excitement of competition and to the cheering crowds in the transition area. But on a purely physiological level, the use of fresh muscles in sprinting toward your bicycle helps offset the accumulated effects of fatigue from the long swim.

Once the cycling leg is complete and the quadriceps muscles roll in tired and fatigued, the same rejuvenating effect occurs in the switch to running.

FASTER RECOVERY

In addition to the natural rejuvenating effect familiar to cross-trainers, switching gears to another activity helps your body perform the vital physiological function of flushing lactic acid from your system. Similar to what occurs during a cooldown after strenuous exercise, during cross-training the lactic acid is flushed into your bloodstream. This helps speed recovery and increases the likelihood of improved performance.

THE CARRYOVER BENEFIT

Although one of the keys to performance is sport-specificity (which we'll discuss soon), there is some carryover benefit from one physical activity to another. (The key word to remember, however, is *some*.)

Certain activities can have some carryover benefit in two different activities. For example, when you run up hills, you are using the vastus lateralis, a portion of your hamstring muscle also used during climbing in cycling. So in this case, the increase in capillary density of this muscle while running up an incline should help your cycling.

There is also some carryover in the type of muscle fiber exercised during cross-training. For example, any physical activity that uses slow-twitch muscles should carry over some benefit to another activity that uses these same types of muscles. (Slow-twitch muscles are those used primarily for endurance sports, such as marathon running. Fast-twitch muscles are those used primarily in sprint situations, such as track and field.)

My dance training has taught me that there are some definite carryover effects from two seemingly unrelated physical activities. Although my participation in triathlon came much later, the strength, flexibility, and kinesthetic coordination I developed during many years in ballet helped me make the transition to endurance sports much more easily.

INJURY PREVENTION

Although injury is certainly a possibility for a multisport athlete or triathlete, training in more than one activity significantly improves your chances of staying healthy. Cross-training distributes the stress of exercise over the entire muscle network. No one muscle group is likely to be taxed beyond its limits.

For example, marathon runners are particularly susceptible to overuse injury because of the constant stress and strain of using the same leg muscles, mile after mile. Increasingly, long-distance runners are integrating a day or two of cross-training into their schedules as both a mental break from pounding the pavement and a method of easing sore leg muscles. Some opt for swimming because it's a nonimpact way of exercising the upper body and gently working out the lower body.

Many runners opt for cycling workouts, an activity that may seem to defeat the purpose of resting tired legs. In actuality, cycling and running work similar muscles but in different ways. This is a classic example of the relationship of muscle groups within the framework of cross-training. During most of the running motion, your hamstrings are contracting. The primary muscle group that contracts during the motion of cycling is the quadriceps. Thus, for the runner who cycles, not only are the cardiovascular benefits of elevating the heart rate achieved, but cycling strengthens muscle groups that would normally be weaker.

And that can give you a healthy respect for a cardinal rule in athletics: wherever you have weakness, that's where you are most susceptible to injury.

MORE REHABILITATION OPTIONS

When injury does occur, cross-training can help maintain your cardiovascular fitness while giving the injured muscle group a chance to rest and heal.

Many runners opt for water-related exercises such as water running. Using a specially designed buoyancy device strapped to your chest, you can mimic the same activity as running. Water running gives you the same aerobic benefits without imposing musculoskeletal strain from the pounding.

CROSS-TRAINING VS. SPORT-SPECIFICITY

Although there are definite crossover benefits from one form of exercise to another, it is a myth that cross-training eliminates the need for sport-specific training. Like most things in life, nothing is guaranteed to work all the time, especially if you don't follow the rules. And one of the fundamental rules of exercise physiology is the principle of sport-specificity. This principle tells you that—while cross-training has definite performance advantages—you can't expect to improve your marathon by spending all your free time in the swimming pool.

Each physical activity is unique and makes different demands on your body. Each form of exercise presents a different set of unique variables and challenges on many different levels: physiologically, biomechanically, even psychologically.

One of the most important variables, particularly to the triathlete, is technique. To remain competitive, triathletes must develop good swim stroke technique, find the most aerodynamic cycling position, and maintain good running form. You can't improve your aerodynamic position in the pool, your stroke on an aero bar, or your running form on your bicycle. Each of these technical skills must be learned by training in the specific activity.

Cross-training is an ideal way to safely develop a solid base of aerobic fitness, which makes it an ideal training approach for the serious fitness enthusiast. But if your goal involves a specific sport, you have to develop the specific muscle groups and skills related to that activity. And for the multisport athlete who is aiming for optimum performances in several different events, a cross-training program must be carefully structured so that each activity is addressed appropriately.

FINDING TIME FOR CROSS-TRAINING

Another common myth is that cross-training requires an extraordinary amount of time. If you're a serious athlete—whether a full-time competitor or weekend warrior—you know the value of time, and usually there isn't much of it. So the fallacy many people buy into is that cross-training takes all day.

On the surface, that outlook makes sense. If you're training for a marathon, married, and working full time, it's hard enough just to get in an early morning or evening run. Your weekly training schedule probably looks like this: (a) you run 6 days out of the week; (b) you run an hour at a time on weekdays; (c) you have one weekly track session; (d) your long, slow distance runs are on weekends. So you ask yourself: How in the world am I going to make time for swimming and biking?

If you're a cyclist, the time commitment is usually much greater. To make significant improvements on the bicycle, multiple long bike rides are necessary during the week, with your shortest ride lasting at least an hour. On weekends, your 100-mi rides or centuries could take you 6 or 7 hr, not including travel time. That's a huge time commitment, so where would you find the time to run or swim?

If you are a single-sport athlete and want to improve your fitness level through cross-training, odds are it can be done with minimal increases in the time you now spend exercising each week. Once you apply the principles in this book, cross-training will become an integral part of your active lifestyle.

But I'd be remiss if I didn't acknowledge that you may need to increase your time commitment. Another alternative is to find new ways of *creating* time, such as cycling back and forth from work, swimming at the health club during your lunch hour, or jogging with your toddler safely strapped in a newly purchased baby stroller.

To be more time-efficient, you'll need to address other relevant performance issues as well; I'll discuss such topics as mental conditioning, nutrition, resting, scheduling, and competition in future chapters.

Smart training methods can also be a big factor in making the best use of your time. An efficient training approach will help you achieve your goals in the minimum amount of time. In the next section, I'll describe a workout method I've used to make the most of my training—and my time.

THE KEY WORKOUT METHOD

I use a training approach to certain workouts that any triathlete or high-level fitness enthusiast who is strapped for time (and who isn't?) would find beneficial. I call them my key workouts, and they are the main component of my cross-training program.

We know that to excel in a specific sport, you have to train in that unique activity. Key workouts are based on the premise that it's just as vital to simulate the conditions of competition (or whatever your method of measuring performance may be). Some of the conditions you need to simulate are pace, terrain, transitions, technical skills, even feedings and hydrating. (What endurance athlete hasn't made the unfortunate mistake of trying a new sports drink or energy bar for the first time on the day of a race? The results are sometimes disastrous and often nauseating.)

I developed the key workout concept over several years, largely by trial and error (but I'd have to say mostly by error). I spent the first 3 years of my triathlon career making mistakes, readjusting my training schedule to fit every new idea or conform to every new training partner. My mileage totals were always changing. The intensity of each workout was never planned. There were some weeks when almost every day was hard, a few when too many were easy. Needless to say, if I had measured my mileage and workout totals on a graph, it would have looked like the world's most dangerous roller coaster.

Although my many training partners adhered to various training philosophies, I noticed a prevalence of mileage junkies during those triathlon pioneering days in San Diego. The variations were tremendous; some pros were averaging 200 mi on the bicycle each week on the low end, with triathletes like Scott Molina topping out at 500 mi. There were a handful of others too—Dave Scott, Mark Allen, Scott Tinley—who could handle and perform well with high-mileage workouts. But for the majority, myself included, there was widespread burnout, injury, and inconsistent performance.

As I watched and trained with the better triathletes, those who consistently raced well and never seemed to be tired or injured, I noticed something common to all of their training regimens. Their focus was not on just being out there and putting in the miles, but on a few particularly intense workouts tailored to simulate their own individual performance goals.

Specifically, the pattern seemed to indicate that one key workout in each of the three events was optimal for triathlon performance enhancement and exercise recovery. I explored the parameters of this new training approach and found that doing more than three of these special sessions per week in each activity didn't give my muscles enough time to recover. One key workout per event provided the optimum balance, although I could sometimes safely stretch it to two or three if I felt my body could adapt. On the down side, I discovered that less than one key workout per event yielded little improvement.

From runners and cyclists who seemed to be using this same method, I learned that two key workouts per week, possibly three, were needed to improve performance in a single sport.

I attribute much of my success in the Gatorade® Ironman Triathlon to the key workout approach. Since I structured my weekly workout program to include at least one key workout in swimming, cycling, and running per week, my performances have been much more consistent and continue to improve. (In chapter 8, we'll discuss key workouts in greater detail.)

CHOOSING THE RIGHT EXERCISE

There are so many popular cardiovascular exercises available to active people that choosing among them may be the hardest part. There are countless activities that will do the job. As long as you increase your heart rate for an extended and sustained period, you are conditioning yourself for endurance.

How do you decide which cross-training activities to choose? First you must recognize that you have to limit your choices. You also have to bear in mind the available resources, such as time, money, and energy. It's better to do two or three things well than to try to master six or seven different physical activities and do a mediocre job at each.

If you have some idea where you want to go and what you want to do, then you probably know which physical activity and which commitment level will take you there. If you have a specific goal, such as competing in a particular event or setting a personal record in a race, obviously you have to concentrate on that sport.

If you are a single-sport athlete using cross-training to supplement your training program, it's easy to let cross-training activities distract you from your main sport. Once you've committed to a specific fitness goal, don't be diverted at a critical juncture in your training. For example, 2 weeks before a marathon is not the time to experiment with in-line skating. Not only is it inappropriate to your training, but you are running the risk of injury, which is always high when you're first learning a technical sport.

Ultimately, your cross-training choices have to align with your unique preferences and lifestyle. You should also give yourself some time away from an activity that you've been participating in for awhile, especially if you've completed a goal. If you've been training for a year to run a marathon, once you've crossed that finish line, give yourself a break for the next 6 months. Try something new. You can still keep running, but go to an aerobics class three times a week or discover the fun of in-line skating. You will not only benefit from a cross-training perspective, but the variety will keep you mentally fresh.

You might call this approach "periodized cross-training," the ultimate method of staying motivated with your fitness regimen. Look at life as a series of cycles, and rotate your exercise activities regularly, introducing new activities as they become evident and as your interests broaden. By doing this, your commitment to fitness will be a rewarding, lifelong experience that will never grow stale and will help you retain your zeal.

Whether you're a single-sport athlete who can't decide which cross-training activities to choose, a triathlete looking for a bit of diversion during the off-season, or a fitness enthusiast looking for new challenges, here's an overview of some of the more demanding cardiovascular exercises, as well as some of my favorites.

RUNNING

One of the best—and most basic—cardiovascular exercise is running because there is almost no one who can't run. It doesn't require a lot of thought, technique, or equipment, which is why running has always been a popular exercise.

Running was my first love, and I've always appreciated its simplicity. Running is very "grounding." I can do it wherever I am, and it allows me to survey new surroundings or explore unfamiliar territory. When I travel, one of the first things I do is go out for a run so I can become familiar with the neighborhood, whether it be a mountain trail or a downtown sidewalk (although I'd prefer a trail to a sidewalk any day).

For you weight watchers, running burns a substantial amount of calories, more than most other forms of exercise. Running also trains your cardiovascular system very quickly because your heart rate is elevated to moderately high levels for a sustained period.

SWIMMING

Swimming is a very complete form of exercise. Although it is muscle-specific, it requires you to use various parts of your body simultaneously. An advantage of swimming is its passive nature. It is a totally non-weight-bearing activity that doesn't impose the stresses on your body that running or cycling do, so injuries are less likely.

Swimming requires substantial athleticism in the areas of aerobic capacity, speed, strength, endurance, flexibility, coordination, and technical skill.

Unfortunately, since most triathletes come from a running background, swimming is commonly a weak event. Also, many triathletes lack an efficient stroke and are uncomfortable in the water. I was fortunate to learn swimming at an early age, but all is not lost if your swimming is not up to par.

Enlist the help of a swimming coach or a swim instructor at a local health club or YMCA. Most local organizations have beginning swimming programs. I know many people who have learned to swim late in life and grown to love it.

Another tip: Being uncomfortable in the water is a major contributor to poor swimming ability. It affects breathing, as well as stroke and kicking skills. If swimming is your weakness, spend time in the pool at least 4 to 6 days a week. Once you're comfortable in the water, swimming can become your favorite workout.

Which brings us to an important point: *always devote more time and energy to your weakness.* Although this may be hard advice to follow, overcoming a weakness can be one of the most gratifying goals you ever achieve.

THREE TRIATHLETES, THREE WEAKNESSES

A perfect example of triathletes making the mistake of ignoring a weakness, as well as concentrating too much on a strength, is played out for me at the same time every year by the same players. My close friends and training partners, Wolfgang Dittrich, Jurgen Zack, and Paul Huddle, are considered three of the best male triathletes in the world. However, each year they continue to make the same training error of ignoring their weakness. (I hope they'll still be my friends after I critique their training habits.)

Germany's Wolfgang Dittrich is a premier swimmer in triathlon and is consistently first out of the ocean at the Gatorade® Ironman World Championship. His cycling is excellent as well and has improved each year. He has often maintained his lead off his bike at the Ironman, dominating two-thirds of this international endurance event. But his Achilles' heel is running. There is nothing more frustrating than leading a race as grueling as the Ironman for so long, only to be passed up on the run. And Wolfgang should know; it's happened to him several times.

Jurgen Zack is another German triathlete and a cycling powerhouse. (He holds the bicycle course record in Hawaii.) The problem is that Jurgen is so far behind the leaders by the time he's finished with the swim, he has to spend most of his energy catching up and doesn't have much left for the run.

American Paul Huddle is one of the finest runners in the sport and among the fastest runners in Hawaii. He's a solid swimmer as well, exiting the water in a respectable position among the pros. But Paul invariably loses his edge on the bike course, falling behind the better cyclists and starting the run with too much of a gap to close.

These otherwise strong triathletes have their obvious weaknesses: Dittrich's is running, Zack's is swimming, and Huddle's is cycling. So after the racing season, what do you suppose they do to hone their abilities during the valuable off-season, a noncompetitive time that is ideal for working on your weakness?

Well, every year Dittrich goes back to Germany to swim competitively in a hometown club, Zack races mountain bikes, and Huddle spends his weekends running road races.

Go figure.

CYCLING

Cycling is a time-consuming activity and requires a significant equipment investment, but the benefits of cycling are virtually unmatched. It is mentally, technically, and physically challenging. It is also an excellent strength conditioner if you live in an area where you are forced to climb steep hills and inclines.

Cycling is a very social sport. Even though there isn't much talking during the intense moments of my Wednesday Rides, there is plenty of banter and socializing during the easy warm-ups and cooldowns.

Perhaps the most exciting aspect of cycling is the speed, which some find intimidating. During my group ride, we average close to 30 mph. On descents, it's common for speeds to reach up to 50 mph. Female athletes seem to be more alarmed by these cycling speeds than their male counterparts. As with swimming, getting comfortable with cycling speed takes patience, persistence, and a lot of hard work. Once you find yourself flying down a mountain road with a big grin on your face, you'll never be afraid of speed again.

MOUNTAIN BIKING

Mountain biking is a fast-growing and popular sport—not just in America but around the world. This is evidenced by the recent inclusion of mountain biking events in the Olympics. (This occurred without the typical demonstration procedure, which usually takes anywhere from 4 to 8 years after application to the Olympic

Committee. This procedure was bypassed with mountain biking, largely because of its tremendous popularity.)

If I had a choice, I would spend less time riding the roadways on my racing bike and more on off-road trails with my mountain bike. In some ways, the cardiovascular workout on a mountain bike is superior to that of a racing bike because of all the climbing and the higher gear turnover. It's also more exciting.

Your geographical surroundings are a lot more interesting, too. Instead of spending hours on a long stretch of lonely roadway (or worse, a crowded stretch of congested streets), you can ride through scenic off-road trails on your mountain bike.

WALKING

I've recently become a big fan of walking, as has the rest of the country. It's a fair cardiovascular workout, a good muscular workout, and an excellent social activity if done with others. You also have time to look around and take in your surroundings, more so than with running and cycling.

If you think that walking is too subdued an activity for a peak fitness program, think again. Walking can be almost as strenuous as running, depending on your pace and the length of your stride. Some racewalkers who compete in walking competitions outwalk the majority of runners. I've seen elite racewalkers complete a marathon in 3 hr, a time most devout marathon runners aspire to.

IN-LINE SKATING

In-line skating is another somewhat technical sport that requires an equipment investment. However, its breakneck speed enables you to cover a lot of ground in an exciting and fun way. Although most advertisers would have you believe it's all fun (which it is), in-line skating is also a demanding cardiovascular workout.

With in-line skating, most of the emphasis is on the lower body—you feel it most in the legs, buttocks, and hips. The pushing-off motion is harder than it looks, but once you've built up enough speed, you'll be hooked.

Cyclists, in particular, have taken to in-line skating as an alternative exercise because it is an excellent workout for your quadriceps muscles. Although different in nature, the technical aspect of the sport and the orientation to speed can also benefit you in cycling.

AEROBICS

Aerobics requires aerobic capacity, coordination, flexibility, and strength. And aerobics has become so varied that you can almost plan your entire peak fitness regime around it.

But until someone comes up with a swim-bike-step-slide-funk format, keep in mind that joining an aerobics class isn't going to improve your triathlon times. Period.

Does that mean you have to miss out on all the excitement? Not at all. Aerobics can be a welcome diversion during racing season or a good off-season activity if you live in an area where you're forced to work out indoors.

"The ideal training is performing the specific sport in similar conditions," says Rob Sleamaker, MS, author of *Serious Training for Serious Athletes*. "But whenever you go indoors to train, you face a motivational problem. Doing something different can make going to the gym fun."

If you think fun is all you're going to have, though, you're in for a surprise—aerobics can drain the fittest Ironman. According to the Institute of Nutrition and Fitness, you'll burn 276 calories during a 30-min step aerobics workout using an 8-in. bench (approximate caloric expenditure for an individual weighing 127-137 lb). That's only slightly less than you burn swimming a mile in the pool.

There are almost as many aerobic trends and techniques as there are Jane Fonda look-alikes. Although step aerobics has been around awhile, it continues to be very popular. The latest trend is Slide, in which you don a pair of special slick booties and slide side to side on a slippery plastic board with bumpers. There's also Funk, which combines traditional aerobics with the latest dance steps and "alternative" music.

Whichever method of madness you choose, aerobics may be a shock to your otherwise injury-proof body, so start slowly and build up to a full workout. Flexibility is especially important with this type of activity, so make sure you supplement your aerobics with a solid stretching program such as the one described in chapter 3.

STAIRCLIMBING

While recovering from my running injury, I used stairclimbing as my transitional tool from water running to the real thing. It allowed my legs to sustain minimal weight-bearing force and gradually become accustomed to the stress while improving my cardiovascular fitness.

Stairclimbers are a relatively new introduction to the health club scene, but no gym would be complete without them. There are several different types of stairclimbers, each mimicking the climbing activity in a different way. The single-action models (StairMaster® and others) work only the legs, and the dual-action models (VersaClimber® and others) add an upper body workout. Some use actual steps that rotate around a belt drive; others use pedals or steppers.

No matter which stairclimber you use, you'll most likely find it an exhaustive workout. Many of the major muscle groups that are key to strong cycling and running performances are used during stairclimbing.

"A lot of triathletes use stairclimbers because it helps both your running and biking," says Ironman colleague Sixto Linares, a top amateur triathlete and spa manager of a downtown Chicago luxury hotel.

When I'm traveling and pressed for time, stairclimbers can provide a quick, high-quality indoor workout. You can get a good, high-intensity workout on a stairclimber in only 20 min.

INDOOR ROWING

There are times when I dread going inside for a workout. Why? The lack of a competitive environment seems to make the time drag. Many health clubs have remedied this by creating indoor competitions and contests.

One of the most organized, worldwide indoor sports is rowing. The competitions are organized by Concept II®, a manufacturer of a flywheel ergometer rower, affectionately known as the "erg" to veteran rowers. The competitions, known as the "Crash-B Sprints," are 2,500 m long—as measured by the erg's electronic board—which is 500 m longer than the Olympic rowing course and is timed to tenths of a second. Very sophisticated stuff.

"I like the competitive aspect," says recently retired professional triathlete Joanne Ritchey, who holds the indoor Crash-B Sprints world record in the women's 30-39 age division. "It's a nice change of pace, something totally different that takes only ten minutes."

Ritchey points out, however, that competing in an indoor rowing competition may be the toughest 10 min of your life. Besides the typical burning sensation in the arms, shoulders, and back, legs are also pushed to the limit.

"Most people don't realize that 75% of rowing is in the legs. I feel the burn most in the gluteals and quadriceps," she says. "I don't know if it helps, but I've had success with triathlons since I started rowing, which means to me that I'm having success with triathlon muscles, not rowing muscles."

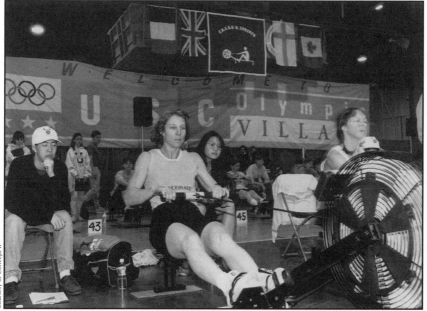

Retired professional triathlete Joanne Ritchey competes in the Concept II Crash B Sprints competition, an international indoor rowing competition.

Even if you don't participate in a competition, rowing can add an extra dimension to your workout. Many rowers are equipped with electronic displays that pit you against a computerized competitor.

"One of the criteria for an off-season program," says Glenn Town, author of *The Science of Triathlon Training and Competition*, "is *not* to bike, *not* to run, *not* to swim. It helps from a mental refreshment perspective."

CROSS-COUNTRY SKIING

If you are looking for a cross-training alternative that is excellent for increasing your aerobic capacity, consider cross-country skiing. It requires a high level of aerobic capacity—cross-country skiers can burn from 600 to 900 calories per hour, with champion athletes burning upwards of a whopping 1,000 calories per hour.

Like swimming, cross-country skiing is a low-impact sport, reducing the possibility of injury. In addition, cross-country skiing works on several different areas of the body simultaneously, giving you a more complete workout.

Still can't decide? In Table 5.1 you'll find a summary of the benefits of several exercises and, if you're a calorie counter, the average expended calories in a 30-min workout.

Table 5.1   Cross-Training Exercises

Activity	Benefits	Calories Burned in 30-min Workout
Running	Excellent cardiovascular conditioner; burns calories fast; great for building lower body muscular strength and endurance	380 (7 mph)
Swimming	Excellent cardiovascular conditioner; nonimpact; increases coordination skills	250 (crawl, 45 yd/min)
Cycling	Excellent cardiovascular conditioner; low impact; great for building lower body muscular strength and endurance; increases technical and coordination skills	240 (low intensity, 12 mph)
Walking	Fair cardiovascular conditioner if done at faster paces; strengthens lower body; allows you to take in surroundings	200 (4.5 mph)
In-line skating	Good cardiovascular conditioner; strengthens lower body; helps you learn better coordination and balance	330 (high intensity)
Aerobics	Excellent cardiovascular conditioner; enhances balance and coordination skills	276 (high intensity)
Stair-climbing	Good cardiovascular conditioner; low impact; good tool for recovery from running injuries	320 (high intensity)
Indoor rowing	Excellent cardiovascular conditioner; low impact; competitions increase enjoyment	330 (high intensity)
Cross-country skiing	Excellent cardiovascular conditioner; low impact; works upper body as well as lower body	330 (high intensity)

Note: These are typical values for people of average size and at a good fitness level. Highly trained athletes can burn substantially more calories per hour.

Sources: *The Athlete Within* by Harvey B. Simon, MD, and Steven R. Levisohn, MD (1987), and *The Encyclopedia of Health: Exercise* by Don Nardo (1992).

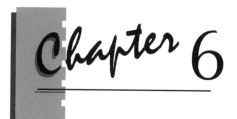

Chapter 6

The Mental Edge

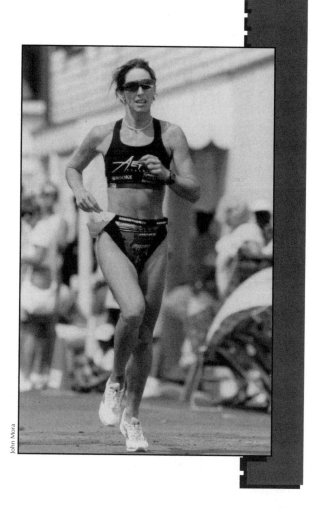

John Mora

There's no doubt that being mentally prepared for a competitive event is important to success in sports. I invest a great deal of energy and time in preparing mentally for an important competition. And not just in the few days preceding the event, but during my entire training period.

However, relying solely on mental techniques as a substitute for solid training is like trying to will your car to run without gas. You can visualize doing the Ironman until you're blue in the face, but if you haven't put in many months of swimming, cycling, and running workouts, chances are you won't finish.

With the understanding that proper training is the base on which you sharpen your mental focus and concentration, in this chapter we'll look at some of the ways you can mentally prepare for a competition and even improve your performance.

TIPS FOR GREATER MENTAL FOCUS AND CONCENTRATION

Let's look at some of the empowering mental attitudes, tools, and techniques I use for focused training and a sharp mental edge during competition. Some are oriented more toward training; some apply specifically to race situations. My experience has taught me that all of them can propel you to perform at your best.

FOCUS ON PERSONAL FITNESS AND PERFORMANCE OBJECTIVES; DON'T COMPARE

There will always be someone to challenge you; that's the nature of competition. But the incessant worries that constant comparisons spawn can quickly suck the energy from your best physical efforts.

Avoid comparing altogether if you can. At first, making comparisons can occur at a subtle, almost undetectable level and will infiltrate your mind like a thin mist. But it can take firm hold of your performance and limit you in the most severe way.

Comparing yourself to others before a race—even to strangers you know nothing about—can become a tough habit to break. And once you've preprogrammed yourself to look upon those you train and race with on a regular basis as superior, once you've slotted yourself as the slow one in the group, you are etching an image in your mind that is not easily erased.

Being careful about how you communicate—both with yourself and with others—is one of the keys to avoiding the comparison trap. Prior to competition, don't communicate with other athletes—even if they're friends—on anything that relates to athletics, anything that may trigger a comparison. Make training and racing a taboo subject.

That's easier said than done if you have friends or competitors who can't seem to talk about anything else. Switch off if you have to. You can interact with them, but don't communicate with them on that level. Abruptly change the subject. Talk about anything else: the latest wedding, somebody's dog, the weather, anything but athletics. Sooner or later, they'll get the picture.

THE PRO COMPARISON GAME

Throughout my career, I've been guilty of playing the comparison game with my professional colleagues. Prior to any major race, a meeting is held for all the professional triathletes to discuss the race course. Many times, the "pro meeting" is my first glimpse at key competitors I may not have seen for months and newcomers to the sport I've never seen before.

As you might imagine, it is tempting to make a few comparisons at these meetings. I've sat at my share of pro meetings looking like I'm paying attention to the race director, when secretly I'm staring at my latest rival. *God, she looks great. She looks fitter than I am.*

When I make comparisons at these meetings, there's usually a snowball effect. The comparisons linger in my mind up to the day of the race. Invariably, I don't do as well as I'd hoped and often find myself beaten by those I've slotted myself below.

Then there are those pro meetings when I walk in and simply acknowledge the presence of other competitors without giving any thought to their fitness level or their training regimen. I don't compare. I hold onto feelings of confidence and think of all the great workouts and performances I've had in the past few months. At those times I am more relaxed in the days prior to a race. I can't honestly say I've always done well when I avoided making comparisons, but those races always seem to be less stressful and more enjoyable.

STRIVE TO MEET YOUR OWN EXPECTATIONS, NOT OTHERS'

Expectations can also be a drain on your mental strength and concentration, especially in the heat of competition. When you create an expectation about the physical outcome of a competition or race—whether it's a finishing time or a ranking—you're setting yourself up for possible disappointment and undue pressure.

If you find it difficult to focus inward and avoid expectations, try looking at things from a different perspective. Come to grips with a startling fact—and I realize how hard this may be to a lot of people who have been taught since childhood that nothing else matters but results. Are you ready?

NO ONE REALLY CARES HOW WELL YOU DO.

Neither your neighbors nor the people at work are going to treat you differently because of what you've done or haven't done on a weekend morning. No one is even going to remember a few weeks later. Realize now, once and for all, that no one cares if you set a personal best. No one except you, of course. Now that isn't such a scary thought, is it?

Changing how we talk to ourselves and the questions we ask ourselves can reduce preoccupation and worry over other people's opinions as well as shatter any outward expectations. If you find it difficult to break away from expectations and focus on inward goals and feelings, examine your inner dialogue. Do you find yourself asking the incessant "what ifs" during racing and competition?

What if I don't finish this race first?

What if I don't place in my age group?

What if I don't finish this 10-km road race in under 40 min?

Next time these questions pop into your mind during competition, don't succumb to the usual worrisome thoughts and crisis-like hysteria. Instead, try the "so what" solution. When you notice the "what ifs" creeping into your head, simply rephrase the question in your mind starting with the words "so what."

So what if I don't finish the race first?

So what if I don't place in my age group?

So what if I don't finish this 10-km road race in under 40 min?

With this turn of phrase worries seem absurd. Everything is put into proper perspective. You realize instantly how silly you've been to put so much energy into such trivial matters.

DO AS I SAY, NOT AS I DO

No matter how firmly I believe in and teach the value of avoiding expectations, I sometimes still fall into that trap. The Zofinger Duathlon in Switzerland is a huge early-season race with extensive media coverage from around the world. It is hotly contested among the pros and has a fairly large prize purse. In the spring of 1993, I was interviewed by a television crew 2 months before the race, and the first question they asked was how I thought I would finish. At the time, my training was going extremely well. I considered myself strong and healthy, as fit and fast as I'd ever felt in my life. I sat there under all the camera lights and—in all my overconfidence—proclaimed that I was in the greatest shape of my life and that I would be going hard from the start.

"Anybody who wants to try and go with me is going to suffer," I smugly proclaimed for all the world to hear. "They may hang on as long as they can, but they're going to be blown off the back."

In my overconfidence, I had blindly succumbed to the expectations trap. What had I done by making that statement? I had created an immense measuring stick for myself among the media, my peers, the whole viewing audience. Can you imagine the pressure when I "toed the line" that morning in Zofinger? Can you imagine what it would feel like to tell the whole world you're going to beat the pants off the competition and then have to prove it?

What happened? Well, I did take off hard—and died a few miles later, finishing a dismal fourth and feeling lousy. It turned out to be a terrible day for me.

What went wrong? In the months following the interview, with this weighty expectation constantly nagging at me, I had overtrained myself to the point of fatigue. I had built myself up as this indestructible and invincible athlete and had lost all rational sense. I thought I could handle the extra training but expected too much of myself. (Had I not created this immense expectation, I believe I would have been more rational and smarter about my training.) As a result, my muscles were overworked and my mind stressed out on the morning of the race. It was a bitter, disappointing experience, and I suffered physically for weeks afterward.

DEVELOP AND USE A PRECOMPETITION RITUAL

I have a peculiar—but effective—ritual that I perform prior to any big race or competition to which I'm traveling. Before boarding the airplane, I allow enough time to stop at the airport terminal bookstore and pick up a bestseller. It doesn't matter what it is. Sometimes it's Robert Ludlum, other times a trashy romance novel—anything I can immerse myself in completely that is altogether detached from the world of professional competition. This may not seem like a mental technique for improving performance, but my absorption in bestsellers has had as much to do with winning the Ironman seven times as anything else.

Although I've never really examined my airport bookstore ritual from a psychological point of view, I suppose the reason it helps me so much is that it serves as a momentary distraction from constant preoccupation with the upcoming race. Reading fiction bestsellers transports me from the world of fast-paced training and competition into one of government conspiracies, erotic romances, and murder mysteries. It's my way of blanking out worrisome thoughts about the future and bringing my mind back to the present (albeit a fictitious one).

In the days preceding a world-class event, I also go on a black-and-white movie binge. I spend hours in front of the set in Hawaii watching old John Wayne or Humphrey Bogart flicks. Although I attend to all the necessary prerace details, such as preparing my equipment—bicycle, running shoes, clothing, once I've done that, I quit worrying about it and immerse myself in the world of classic films.

My prerace bestseller and movie fests help me to stand on the beach prior to a triathlon with a fresh and energetic mind. Removing myself from worry about the future—even for a few days—has helped me to gain a foothold on the present. My thinking is clear and my mind is focused and relaxed.

There are, of course, those competitors who do nothing but fret about the future. They call it preparation. I call it needless worry. For example, unlike many professional runners and triathletes, I don't do a detailed prerace survey of the course. I may ride or run the course, just to get a feel for it, but I don't worry about such minor details as the gravel on the beach or a pothole on the cycling course. I trust myself to deal with them during the race in the best way possible.

For me, thinking and worrying about the future takes a tremendous amount of energy. I've learned to relax largely because I am incapable of dealing with the stress of thinking too much about a race. In the past, it literally drove me crazy, resulting in major stress symptoms such as excessive nervousness and vomiting.

You may never have to deal with the pressures of professional competition, but if you've ever committed yourself to training for an important event, you know how it feels to be overwhelmed.

Create a prerace ritual that takes your mind off the energy-draining, stress-inducing worries about an upcoming race. Think of some of the things you've always wanted to waste time on but have been too preoccupied with the reality of competition to do it. Perhaps, like me, you'd like to read a trashy novel or watch old movies. Maybe you'd like to do some socializing, visit some non-athletic friends who won't know the difference between an aero bar and a PowerBar®. How about a walk in the park or on the beach? A Saturday afternoon nap on a hammock? A game of pinball?

If you've done your homework (and even if you haven't), don't be afraid to take a time-out prior to racing to do something far removed from the sport. The rewards will be a fresher perspective and a state of mind focused on the present.

ESTABLISH A MENTAL PROGRAM FOR PERFORMANCE

People frequently ask me what I'm thinking about when I'm racing. They often comment that I seem so relaxed, yet determined. I am totally focused on my body during competition. I am constantly checking every technical aspect of my performance—the efficiency of my swim stroke, my rpm's during cycling, my leg turnover on the run, my nutritional requirements. In a race like the Ironman, you can't go very far before running out of fuel, so I'm constantly checking energy levels and monitoring fluid and solid food intake.

How can I be monitoring all that? Do I run with a portable laptop computer strapped to my back? The human body has a remarkable ability to monitor itself, and that is the key in competition. Focus on your body—every single aspect that relates to the efficient use of your muscles and the energy available to them—and you'll find you're built very much like a computer.

Computers don't worry about whether they're going to perform. They just do. (Or sometimes they just don't—but they don't worry about that either.) Computers are always in a present state of mind. (How else would they get so much done?)

If focusing on precise physiology is something you've never tried, start off slowly. By mentally focusing on one aspect of your exercise, one workout at a time, you'll condition your body to go on automatic.

Eventually, you will be able to monitor every important physiological aspect of your exercise simultaneously—something even the most advanced computers in the world would have a hard time doing.

During your next cycling workout, concentrate on one aspect of your motion. For example, decide to concentrate solely on your pedaling motion and on using your legs in a fluid, even motion throughout the entire 360-deg circle. Picture a perfect circular pedaling motion in your mind. Concentrate on a weak point for many runners and triathletes—the last 180 deg, where you're using more of the hamstring and gluteus muscles. It may seem cumbersome and tedious at first, but if you keep at it, you will start to feel smoother and faster on the bicycle.

Apply this technique to other aspects of your training, remembering to keep your mental focus on something very specific and tangible.

ZONE IN, NOT OUT

While it's important to focus inward while training, it's even more crucial during a competitive event. Many athletes have made the mistake of "zoning out" and disappearing into "the hole" in all the excitement of competition.

They forget to monitor fluid and nutritional needs. They don't eat or drink, and then wonder why they smash into "the wall." As powerful as the mind is, when your muscles are out of glycogen because you haven't taken in carbohydrates, you're not going to be able to finish. (We'll discuss nutrition in greater detail in the next chapter.)

Zoning out can also negatively affect your pace. During the drama and excitement of competition, it's easy to go too hard in the early stages of a race and compete above your head. The adrenaline is pumping and you're not thinking about what's happening to your body. In the later stages, when you find yourself running low on energy, you will wish you had kept a steady, more consistent pace.

DON'T WORRY, BE HAPPY

During training, competition, and afterward, make it a habit to think about your positive feelings about working out. What do you thrive on? What about training makes you feel good? What did you do during a race that you feel proud of?

It only makes sense to focus on making yourself happy at a race, on coming home feeling proud that you put in your best effort, whatever that may mean to you. At the end of a day, perhaps on a Sunday night after a competition when you're winding down and thinking about the events of the day, you alone will have to be happy with yourself.

That could mean many things. You could be happy with yourself for climbing a hill strongly. You could feel happy about sticking with a group of people you'd never thought you'd be able to stay with. Maybe you couldn't stick with them for long, but are happy (and excited) about the challenge this presents for the future. These are the sorts of things I thrive on.

LEAVE YOUR WATCH AT HOME

In the races where I've done the best, many of which have been in Hawaii, there's no better way to describe how it felt than to say it felt effortless. People are invariably astonished when I say this. "How can you swim, cycle, and run for nine hours under sizzling temperatures and dizzying crosswinds and call it 'effortless'?"

Although my "effortless" races are the result of many factors, I avoid one common distraction by leaving my watch at home. I'm not interested in my split after the swim, bike, or run. I'm going out there for the feeling, and my mind is relaxed and free of expectations. I may be out there for 9 hr, but sometimes it feels like 90 min. Measurements of time and place mean nothing to me. Someone in the transition area may say, "Oh, the leader is two minutes ahead." But in my mind, they may as well have said, "Oh, the sun is shining."

Because I refuse to be ruled by the clock, the mental hardship associated with endurance exercise is minimized.

MENTAL TECHNIQUES

In addition to the tips I've just mentioned, two widely accepted techniques that can be used in a variety of situations deserve special attention: visualization and affirmation.

VISUALIZE YOUR WAY TO SUCCESS

Using visualization to improve performance is a mental technique I employ on a regular basis. But unlike many athletes and sports psychologists who may recommend a separate agenda for mental work, I think the most effective way to prepare mentally for a race or competition is to rehearse the race during your training sessions.

For those unfamiliar with the term *visualization*, it can be defined as mental rehearsal. You visualize the ideal goal being fulfilled in your mind before the actual event. By rehearsing the event in your mind as you would like it to occur, you lessen the intimidation, and more importantly, you closely associate yourself with what you'd like to have occur.

As with any mental technique, be very specific about what you visualize. Stay away from visualizing outward expectations and focus instead on the physical manifestation of your inward goals.

For example, if you're a triathlete, visualize how you will look when you're feeling good on your bicycle. See yourself in a relaxed, aerodynamic position, feeling strong, pedaling effectively and precisely. What will that look like? Visualize it in your mind with as much color, emotion, and vivid reality as you can conjure up.

Link your visualization to your exercise. It's fine to sit on your sofa and visualize yourself crossing that in-line skating race finish line first to the cheers of adoring fans, but visualization isn't effective unless you link your mental pictures to exercise and motion. The reality of physical discomfort and effort during a race can easily reverse any mental work you've done away from the training environment.

Training, by itself, is a form of visualization. While doing the physical work, you are training your mind at the same time to deal effectively with the discomfort associated with exercise. When you're on the track doing an interval workout, and you're running fast and feeling good, tune in to that feeling and visualize yourself feeling that way during an upcoming race.

AFFIRM FOR GREATER PERFORMANCE

Affirmations are positive statements you repeat to yourself over and over to effect change and to reinforce desired behaviors and performance. I look at affirmations as personal counseling that can be a strong positive reinforcement for change.

Often when you try to change something in your life, you'll encounter resistance from other people, particularly those who have invested a great deal of time in shaping your behavior. Often you'll find those around you uncomfortable with the concept of change, bombarding you with negative affirmations:

"*You're* not a good swimmer."

"*You're* too scared to swim in open water."

"You're not a very good cyclist."

"You're a very slow runner."

Affirmations are simply a way of countermanding the constant negative affirmations that come at us daily. There are three simple "P" rules when formulating your own personal affirmations: they must be present tense, positive, and personal. Some examples:

"I am a good swimmer."

"I love to swim in open water."

"I am an excellent cyclist."

"I am a fast runner."

Affirmations can be used to strengthen an area of weakness in your fitness regimen or to raise your level of performance a notch higher. Decide on one affirmation a week and repeat it over and over to yourself.

An effective way to use affirmations during training is to condition yourself to repeat them mentally with every other breath or every other stroke, pedal, or stride. How many times should you repeat them? A thousand times a day wouldn't be too many.

The key to affirmations is repetition. Don't be discouraged if your mind seems to be battling with itself and rejecting the affirmation as false or unbelievable. This is due to all the years of garbage clogging your mental pipes. If you're persistent, your affirmations will eventually act like a Roto-Rooter and flush all the limiting debris out of your system. With repeated present-tense, positive, personal affirming, you'll start to believe in your self-worth and act upon those beliefs.

WHO ME? A PURPLE PIG!?

If you look at your life as a script, you might be surprised to find just how much of your script has been written by other people. So much of the way we feel about ourselves comes from the projections (the scripts) we have received from those around us.

In her book *You Can Heal Your Life,* author Louise Hay sets an absurd but thought-provoking scenario: Say you had a close friend who constantly stated, over and over again, "You are a purple pig." What do you think you would do? Chances are you'd eventually tell your friend to shut up, and if the harassment continued, you might get as far away as possible.

Why, then, Hay asks, don't we turn around and reject someone who tells us that we can't be who we want to be or do what we want to do? It's just as ludicrous for someone to say, "You are not a swimmer" or "You are not a triathlete." Spend a few moments thinking back on all the "can'ts" you have heard over the years and how they have affected your life.

Resolve now to write your own script. Begin with the small things, perhaps some nagging negative statements that you hear daily or that have become part of your own inner chatter. Catch them before they sink in. Refuse to accept them anymore. And—if you have to—let others know you don't want to hear them anymore.

Chapter 7

Resting, Recovering, and Eating Right

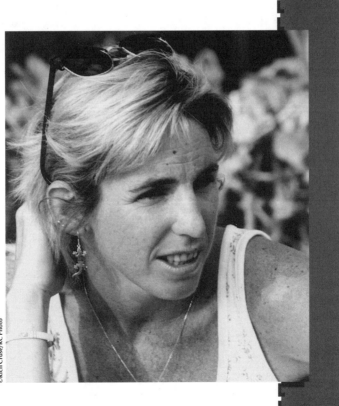

Throughout my years of professional competition, I've found that many seemingly unrelated factors affect athletic performance off the field of play. These include giving yourself enough rest between workouts, helping your body recover with massage therapy, and of course, eating the right kinds and amounts of food.

Although each of these topics is a book-length subject, this chapter will cover some of the fundamentals that affect peak fitness. Much of this chapter is devoted to the fascinating, though complex, topic of nutrition for the female athlete. But just as relevant to your athletic performance is the ability to monitor your body and allow it enough rest and recovery time.

THE BALANCED APPROACH

Rest is perhaps the hardest thing for an athlete to do. That may sound ironic, but the large number of articles and books written on sports injuries clearly shows that athletes and physically active people have a hard time dealing with rest.

Runners are particularly notorious for overdoing it. In *The Runner's Complete Medical Guide*, the authors address the irony of running injuries: "Runners are the fittest group of sick and injured people in the world. While running is probably the most natural and healthful sport ever played, its participants most frequently push their mental and physical capacities to the limit."

Because most triathletes come from a running background, they have their share of running-related injuries. Triathletes have the same overuse tendency as runners, and in the early days of triathlon, the "more is always better" attitude was the norm. Since then, professional runners, as well as triathletes, have learned more about their bodies—quite a bit more. As a result, there is less tendency among those at the professional level to *overtrain*, a term used to describe overuse.

This more balanced approach to fitness has spilled over into traditional sports such as cycling and new activities such as in-line skating and beach volleyball. Examples of this are the increased reliance on massage therapy and proper nutrition and the reduced emphasis on back-to-back hard workouts in these sports.

Most sports injuries result from not allowing the body enough rest and recovery time. I have made it a point to keep the importance of rest foremost in my mind. Because of this, I've managed to stay relatively free of major injury throughout most of my triathlon career. It has only been during those times when rest *wasn't* foremost in my mind that I have paid dearly for it with injury.

Planning and following a wise and effective training schedule that builds in rest days and easy training days for recovery is crucial to avoiding injury, a topic we'll cover in greater detail in chapter 8. But first, it's worthwhile to cover some principles and topics that can help you know when you need rest. If you absorb some of the fundamental knowledge in the following sections, you won't ever have to buy a book or read a magazine article on sports injuries.

STRESS MANAGEMENT

When Mark Allen surged in the final miles of the 1989 Ironman Triathlon and wrestled the lead away from a seemingly invincible Dave Scott, the triathlon world marveled at the resiliency and persistence of the new Kona champion. There had been many previous years when he had failed to take the crown away from Scott. Several times his losses were due to dehydration; one year, it was a series of flat tires. Yet nothing diminished his will to succeed. He came back year after year and persistently strived to win at Ironman until he finally achieved his goal in 1989. However, for many professional triathletes as well as those who worked closely with Allen, what happened on those lava beds that year was an eventuality.

"Mark possesses an exquisite attitude towards training," says Dr. Darryl Hobson, Allen's physician and sports performance specialist. "He never overtrains." Professional triathlete Todd Jacobs agrees: "Mark is such a good example of overall life balance. He's incredibly wired into his body, with nothing lost on him in terms of biofeedback. I think he can tell if there's a vitamin deficiency," he muses.

Allen is the consummate 90s athlete. Everything he says in relation to rest and injury implies a keen body awareness. "The first step is prevention," he notes. "In my mind I am constantly gauging the status of my body, where it needs energy."

Demanding exercise routines and, in particular, endurance sports make constant monitoring of the body an absolute necessity. "Listen to your body" becomes a divine commandment when applied to training for a high level of fitness, with injury the price most often paid for disobedience.

Most experts agree that establishing when the body needs rest affects the ability of an athlete to avoid overtraining, the source of most injury. Yet, with all the internal variables (not to mention external variables such as equipment fit, technique, terrain, etc.), how can one go about establishing a balance, a biofeedback line, as Allen seems to possess? Just exactly how do you listen to your body?

If you think about it, exercise is a stressful activity. A high level of exercise places great demands on the body, and it responds by instinctively increasing its capacity for stress. By taking a look at how the body manages stress, clues may surface that can help you to know when your body needs rest.

THE BODY'S "REST-O-METER"

The body manages stress in many ways. One way is through processes that occur in the autonomic nervous system. This complex system often mediates the response of the body to stress, playing major roles in speeding up heart rate, increasing blood pressure, and mobilizing energy reserves. When your body is taxed beyond healthy levels, the sympathetic nervous system gets a little out of whack, producing some tangible symptoms. Look at the following list of conditions as overtraining signals, or the body's natural Rest-O-Meter, with a well-defined red line.

- Inconsistent episodes of blurred vision and a feeling of eyestrain and sensitivity.
- Varying degrees of joint pain, particularly in the vulnerable sacroiliac (lower back) and knee.
- Muscle weakness, particularly in the calf and medial (inside) of the knee.
- Getting sick easily with slow recovery. Athletes who partake in long or intense exercise tend to have weakened immune systems.
- Allergic reactions. Since a weakened immune system fails to adapt to changes in the environment, athletes who travel frequently experience this problem.
- Insomnia. A biochemical imbalance often throws the body into a state of chaos and "mini-frenzy," resulting in the inability to relax and subsequent loss of sleep.
- Poor digestion. Stress hormones are strongly linked to digestive processes, with severely high levels leading to ulcers and other gastric problems.
- Excessive nervousness and irritability. Although still a subject of much research, overtraining appears to have detrimental effects on psychological behavior.

- Lack of energy, with no reserve energy to surge in the latter half of a workout.

These signals may be indications of a need for rest and possible forthcoming injury, but only experience will draw out the strongest, most dependable warning signs. Each body has its own individual composition and weaknesses. Through the years, I've learned to put more stock in certain signals that tell me I need rest and to ignore others that are less reliable. What's reliable for me, however, may not be for you, and vice versa.

RECOVERING WITH MASSAGE

Massage, or "sports massage" as it applies to the specific needs of the athlete, is a vital hands-on therapy for recovering faster from workouts. Like flexibility training, massage is a much-neglected part of many serious exercise regimens. Some endurance athletes feel that the need for massage is negligible because their particular sport works their body in a specific range of motion. They often conclude that unless that range of motion is impaired, there's no need for massage.

The informed and knowledgeable active person seeking peak fitness knows the value of a once-a-week massage session (twice if you can afford it) with a certified therapist. Here is a short list of some of the tangible physical benefits of massage.

Improves Performance

During exercise, tiny muscle tears occur that need time to heal. The faster you can heal after a workout, the sooner you can start the next one safely. Massage speeds the recovery process from workout to workout by removing the by-products (lactic acid) from muscles.

Improves Awareness

Massage therapy can help you develop a better awareness of your muscles and connective tissue. It can help you learn the subtle differences between normal muscle soreness and the pain of an injury in its early stages.

Promotes Flexibility

During both strength and endurance training, the repeated muscle contractions induce microtrauma in muscle tissue, which may cause adhesions to form. This is perceived as tightness in the muscles.

Massage makes the muscles and tissues more pliable, promoting greater flexibility and more resiliency as well as better circulation.

Gives You Feedback

The most important benefit of massage is the ability of a therapist trained in sports massage to determine areas of weakness or excessive stress that could lead to injury. During my training, particularly during intense periods, the effects of "runner's high" often block my awareness of forthcoming injury. Massage is a "feedback loop" between myself and my muscles. My massage therapist sometimes gives me clues that suggest the possibility of minor injuries, barely discernible damage that could become more serious.

Helps You Heal

Special massage techniques can be used to speed the healing process if you become injured. This can be particularly helpful for overuse injuries. Injured areas need a healthy blood supply to aid the healing process, and massage can help improve circulation in the injured area.

NUTRITION FUNDAMENTALS

During my injury rehabilitation last year, I thoroughly reassessed my diet. I wondered if I could make any nutritional changes that would help my rehabilitation and renew by body from the inside.

Throughout most of my professional career, I'd taken the middle road with regard to nutrition. My motto was "everything in moderation." I reasoned that if I just stuck to that credo, everything would balance out in the end. I didn't eat too much of one kind of food and checked myself when my diet habits went astray.

Because of my injury, I was forced to take a hard look at every possible avenue of improvement. I was also intrigued by the concept of foods playing a significant part in my recovery. So I began to learn and study the fundamentals of nutrition, and I have come to believe that the foods we eat influence performance more than most athletes think. I realized that summer that I couldn't afford to take the middle road anymore. I had to find the optimum diet and eating habits that would add to, not detract from, my training and racing.

In the rest of this chapter, we'll talk about the unique nutritional needs of the active female. Because I'm not a certified nutritionist, I've enlisted the help of researchers and experts in the field of nutrition, including Monique Ryan, a registered dietitian and nutrition consultant specializing in sports nutrition. She has advised me on nutrition facts regarding carbohydrates for training, recovery, and competition, as well as on some interesting studies on protein requirements. Monique has worked with several professional athletes and teams like the Saturn Cycling Team. Together, we'll cover some fundamental nutritional facts that every active woman should know.

NUTRITION AND WOMEN

You are probably aware that, as a woman, you have a greater need for magnesium, calcium, and iron. As an athlete or active female, this need takes on even more significance. I've included a brief summary of these three minerals, but you should consult a nutritionist who specializes in working with athletes for more specific information and recommendations.

Magnesium

Magnesium plays an integral part in the normal functioning of an active woman's body. Magnesium helps convert glycogen to energy, aids in the development and functioning of muscles, and regulates heart rate and blood pressure.

Research has shown that strenuous activities, such as marathon running and cross-country skiing, tend to lower the levels of magnesium in female athletes. In addition, this effect can linger for extended periods, causing potentially serious depletion of magnesium in muscle tissue as a result of frequent or intense exercise.

The National Research Council has set the Recommended Dietary Allowances (RDA) for magnesium at 280 to 350 mg for adult women, although some studies have indicated that higher amounts may be needed for women engaged in regular, strenuous exercise.

The best natural sources of magnesium are whole-grain breads and cereals, nuts, legumes, soybeans, and seafood.

Calcium

Calcium is vital to the athletic female because it is a major component of bones. The need for calcium starts when you're young, and if you get enough calcium early in life, you build a "calcium bank" that can keep your bones strong. Unfortunately, women are at a disadvantage early in life compared to men because they begin with less bone mass.

When your diet is deficient in calcium, this vital mineral is taken from this "calcium bank" supply and used for other normal body functions that require it. This can weaken your bones and increase your likelihood of developing osteoporosis later in life.

Calcium performs other vital functions, such as facilitating the production of hormones and the stimulation of enzymes, and has been linked to combatting stress.

Calcium, along with some other vital minerals, is lost in perspiration. It has been speculated that muscle cramps may be associated with deficiencies of calcium (as well as magnesium, potassium, sodium, and fluid). Keep adequate amounts of these minerals in your diet. For competition and training in hot weather, an electrolyte-containing sports drink may be beneficial. You might want to try using one, especially if you find yourself cramping frequently during exercise.

By performing weight-bearing exercises, such as running, in-line skating, skiing, cycling, dancing, weight-training, or walking, you're already increasing your chances of avoiding osteoporosis. Studies have shown that such activities increase bone mass and help women avoid osteoporosis, something to consider if you're a masters athlete.

The RDA for calcium is 1,200 mg for young adult females and 800 mg for adult females age 25 and older. If you're an athletic female who participates in sports that put stress on your bones, you may want to use the 1,200-mg guideline.

Good sources of calcium include low-fat dairy products, almonds, broccoli, kale, salmon, sardines, spinach, and dried peas and beans. The best-absorbed sources of calcium are low-fat dairy products, such as low-fat yogurt and skim milk.

Iron

Iron carries oxygen to the blood, so without it you wouldn't be able to live. Iron is linked to the hemoglobin in red blood cells, the proper functioning of muscles, and the enzymes associated with energy release. So, as you might guess, such a vital nutrient is essential to an active woman's diet.

Iron deficiency may cause certain types of anemia, which can hinder athletic performance. Sports anemia, a condition that is common among endurance athletes with strenuous training regimens and poor diets, can result from iron deficiency. Nutritionists recommend that women be tested for iron deficiency before beginning any new exercise program. The RDA for iron is 18 mg for women but should be increased to 30 mg or more if you're pregnant.

The best-absorbed sources of iron include lean red meat, turkey, and chicken. Plant sources (not as well absorbed) include egg yolks, raisins, prunes, apricots, dates, leafy green vegetables, dried beans, and figs. Iron-fortified cereals also can help meet your requirements.

THE CARBOHYDRATE CONNECTION

You're probably familiar with three nutrients that come from food: carbohydrate, protein, and fat. Most athletes know that carbohydrate is the most important, though least abundant, fuel for energy. This is because carbohydrate is burned more efficiently than protein or fat. Studies have shown that the energy from carbohydrate can be released within exercising muscles up to three times as fast as the energy from fat.

It's generally accepted that at least 60% to 70% of the calories in an active person's diet should be from carbohydrate. Rice, pasta, cereals, fruits, dried peas and beans, potatoes, vegetables, and whole-grains bread are examples of foods high in complex carbohydrate. Supplements containing both simple and complex carbohydrates are available that can be used as effective nutrition aids to help you meet your high-carbohydrate goals (which we'll discuss later). But the bulk of your diet should come from fruits, grains, and vegetables.

Carbo Loading for Competition

The idea behind carbohydrate loading is simple. Carbohydrate is the best source of glycogen, a clean-burning fuel ideally suited for high-energy efforts. The problem is that—like a gas tank in a car—our muscles can only hold so much glycogen before they run dry. We can store carbohydrate in the form of glycogen, but unfortunately, our capacity is very limited; experts say that after about 2 hr of endurance exercise, liver and muscle glycogen becomes depleted, particularly at high intensities.

For example, about 20 mi into a marathon, you may "hit the wall" or, more descriptively, feel like a Mack truck flattened you. You may experience loss of energy and overwhelming fatigue, nausea, and any number of other unpleasant symptoms, depending on your body's unique physiology.

If you're cycling, perhaps doing a long ride, you may experience a drop in blood glucose levels, a phenomenon known as "bonking." It feels just like it sounds. Your tongue might be hanging over your handlebar, and if you haven't gotten enough liquids, the inside of your mouth might feel fur-lined.

Exercise physiologist Michael Sherman, PhD, of the Ohio State University provides the technical explanation of what's happening here: "When athletes undertake prolonged endurance exercise they deplete glycogen stores that are used for muscle contraction. If you run out of fuel, muscle contraction is impaired and you have to reduce your exercise intensity or stop."

Thus, the purpose of carbohydrate loading is to offset (and possibly avoid) such occurrences in events lasting over 2 hr. In effect, you are trying to create a bigger gas tank, a greater reserve of glycogen to delay running on fumes.

The traditional method of carbohydrate loading, used in the 70s by many marathon runners, is a complicated and controversial technique. Instead, here are two safer and simpler approaches to carbohydrate loading in the week before an event.

1. The first approach is simple: if you're training regularly and eating a high-carb diet, just keep doing what you're doing because you're already carbohydrate loading. (That was easy, huh?) The process of pushing your body harder and harder every day—with proper rest and recovery—actually increases the capacity of your muscles to hold glycogen reserves. You must be consuming the typical athlete's diet of 60% to 70% carbohydrate daily to have this effect.

However, there is a limit to how much you can increase glycogen capacity simply by training and eating right. You will eventually get to the point where, if you want that extra edge, a certain amount of sophisticated dietary manipulation will be necessary.

2. The second approach is most common among marathoners and endurance athletes. Three to 4 days before an event, increase your carbohydrate intake and decrease your training in both intensity and distance.

If you're already on a high-carbohydrate, low-fat diet, it might be difficult to increase your ingestion of carbohydrate. A simple solution is to use one of the high-carbohydrate supplements that are available.

PROTEIN PRINCIPLES

The principal role of protein is to build and repair body tissues, including muscles, ligaments, and tendons. This nutrient also plays a part in the production of enzymes and hormones, thus serving a regulatory function. Proteins are composed of individual units called amino acids. There are 20 amino acids, 11 of which are manufactured by the body. The other 9 are essential amino acids that must be ingested in the foods we eat. If essential amino acids are not consumed, the body's ability to produce certain proteins will be impaired and health and performance may suffer.

According to recent studies, endurance athletes appear to need more protein than the average person. The type of exercise you perform may affect amino acid turnover and may dictate protein requirements. Endurance exercise increases amino acid oxidation (breakdown). Resistance exercise enhances protein turnover and muscle synthesis; therefore, both cardiovascular and strength training exercise increases protein requirements for female athletes.

In a recent study reported in *VeloNews*, Gail Butterfield, PhD, of the Palo Alto Veterans Affairs Medical Centers in California looked at the protein requirements of athletes undergoing strength training. Her research suggests that athletes participating in a moderate to intense strength training program seem to have slightly higher protein requirements. A protein intake of 1.2 to 1.3 g per kilogram of body weight should be adequate. (To determine your body weight in kilograms, divide your weight in pounds by 2.2.) The sedentary person requires 0.8 g of protein per kilogram of body weight per day.

Female athletes at risk for protein deficiency are those who eat excessive amounts of high-carbohydrate foods containing little or no protein. This can also occur in a diet that typically avoids fatty foods. Diets that contain low- or no-fat dairy products, lean meats and poultry, and generous portions of dried peas and beans can provide high-quality protein with less fat. Some active women take protein or amino acid supplements, but elevated nutritional needs are easily met with a well-balanced diet containing adequate amounts of calories.

THE FEAR OF FAT

Many fit women have a conditioned response to fatty foods—they run away from them as if those foods were the plague. But fat isn't all bad; it does serve a vital function in the body. Fat provides a form of stored energy, contributes to healthy skin, and is part of the structure of many hormones and cell membranes. Fat is also a source of the fat-soluble vitamins: A, D, E, and K.

Many active women abhor the fat on their abdomens, but maybe they'd feel better knowing that fat cushions and protects delicate internal organs, such as the kidneys and liver. Fat even performs a life-saving function by helping the body form blood clots that stop bleeding. Active females with below-normal body fat are likely to experience a disruption in their menstrual cycle and a related loss of calcium, making them more prone to stress fractures.

Does that mean you should chuck the boxes of spaghetti and head for the ice cream section at your grocery store? I don't think so. First, consider that fat is a very concentrated source of energy, so small amounts provide many calories and can lead to weight gain and obesity. Second, a high-fat diet has been shown to contribute to the development of heart disease and certain types of cancer. Studies show that chronic diseases related to high fat intake are associated with 2 of the 10 leading causes of death in the United States.

Most nutritionists promote a reduction of fat in the American diet— from the current 37% to 40% of total calories from fat for the average American to fewer than 30%, as the new FDA guidelines on food labels recommend.

WOMEN AND THE WEIGHT ISSUE

In our society, the way we perceive the ideal female body has taken its toll on every woman at one point or another. All too often, weight is the issue that is foremost in our minds. Among active women and female athletes, weight concerns are prevalent, in some ways more than in the mainstream.

The ideal endurance athlete is often seen as having low body fat; the perfect runner, cyclist, or triathlete is perceived to be "lean and mean." Thus, many active women striving for a high level of fitness make the mistake of trying to emulate their lean male counterparts and struggle to lower their body fat through quick-fix weight programs and crash diets. Here are some sound arguments for why that approach is flawed.

Women Are Supposed to Have More Fat

Women don't realize that the female body is designed to store more body fat. Both men and women have about 3%-5% of the essential body fat needed for normal functioning of the body, but women have an additional 5%-8% sex-specific body fat stored in their breasts, thighs, hips, and inner legs.

These fat stores that the female body is "cursed" with are intended for the needs inherent in childbearing. The athletic female who is interested in faster times or greater performance (and not so much in childbearing) may feel frustrated by this fact, but there's no reason to be, as discussed in the following paragraphs.

Thinner May Not Be Better

There's no real proof that the lighter female athlete is better suited for athletics. An example of this is runner Lisa Weidenbach, who has run several sub-2:30 marathons and has won many major races, including Chicago and the Twin Cities. Although the ideal marathon runner is often perceived to be as thin as a rail, Lisa has a natural, normal body type that's bigger than most of her counterparts. Yet she often leaves her competitors in the dust.

In some sports, extra body fat is beneficial. In open-water swimming, body fat helps female athletes stay warmer and more buoyant. Shelley Taylor-Smith has won the mixed-sex 22.5-mi Atlantic City Marathon swim twice, and American Penny Dean swam the English Channel in an amazing 7 hr 40 min, a time no woman *or man* has beaten since.

Weight Is All in the Family

Your weight may not be just a function of your willpower; there are genetic factors involved. Just as it makes no sense to fret over being short or tall, which is also a result of genetics, it makes no sense to frustrate yourself over your natural weight. If you come from a family with a large body type, your normal, natural body type is likely to be similar.

Food Is Fuel

Everyone needs to eat healthy, nutritious foods, but this is especially true for the active woman or female athlete. The foods you eat affect your energy level, your immunity to disease, and even your level of concentration. Exercise places nutritional demands on your body that need to be met with the calories in a balanced diet.

Many active women cut down on their caloric intake at the expense of meeting their unique nutritional needs. As a result, they may lose a few pounds, but their performance often suffers. In addition, a subpar caloric intake could make them more susceptible to injuries and illness.

You may not yet be convinced, but if you attempt to reach an unnaturally low weight by crash dieting or fasting unhealthily, your nutritional deficiencies could hurt your performance, not help it.

A SENSITIVE TOPIC

During my years in endurance sports, I've seen a definite increase in eating disorders among female triathletes. I admit to sometimes being preoccupied with my weight, but there are some athletes who go far beyond normal preoccupation. They become obsessed with weight loss and subsequently deny themselves even the smallest amount of food. This constant conflict with food can be a hellish way to live and will literally destroy your physical and mental health.

Eating disorders such as anorexia nervosa and bulimia seem to be on the rise among female endurance athletes, particularly those at the collegiate level. This is a complex issue, particularly for female athletes, and one that's too big to tackle here. It is best to address such concerns with a professional counselor who specializes in eating disorders and a nutritionist who will help guide you to make proper diet choices.

FLUID FACTS

Fluid replacement is vital to any athlete, particularly those working outdoors at a high level of intensity in warm climates. Here's what happens to your body during that long summer bike ride or sweltering marathon run.

During hard exercise, the amount of heat produced in your working muscles is 15 to 20 times greater than at rest. When your brain is alerted to a rise in body temperature, it sends more blood to the skin, which stimulates sweat. The evaporation of sweat has a cooling effect on your body, but during hard exercise, this evaporation may not be sufficient, causing you to overheat to temperatures above 104°F. In addition, the fluid loss from sweating causes a loss of body weight, medically known as dehydration.

Severe dehydration will result in a decrease in sweating capacity and further increase the possibility of injuries such as heat stroke (which may result in death), heat exhaustion (which will cause excessive tiredness), and muscle cramping (which will spoil your chances of setting a new PR).

Essentially, your heart has to work harder to maintain proper blood flow, and during vigorous exercise, you can become dehydrated in as little as 30 min. While sweating helps, most of us don't sweat efficiently enough to cool our bodies properly. Common sense tells us that the key to avoiding dehydration and other fluid loss injuries is simple; the closer you can come to replacing water loss during exercise, the better off you'll be.

In a demanding event such as the Gatorade® Ironman Triathlon, participants lose approximately 1 to 8 gal of body fluids. This can translate into a weight loss of 5 to 20 lb. Most triathlons don't approximate the weather and course conditions of the Kona event, but timely hydration to replace those lost fluids is essential.

Whether you should use water or a carbohydrate replacement drink to stay properly hydrated depends largely on the duration of exercise. It is generally accepted that water is sufficient for activities lasting less than 90 min, with proper hydration the primary concern.

Sports Drinks

Sports drink companies often purport to have a magic formula, implying that their particular blend of high-tech ingredients can take more time off your 40-km bike leg than aero bars. The reality is that most sports drinks are effective for replenishment of fluids and carbohydrate.

There are some criteria that may narrow your choice. If your mouth puckers and your taste buds scream for mercy, you're less likely to drink enough of what you need. Studies have shown the importance of a pleasing taste for encouraging timely feeding.

Drink 4 to 8 oz of a sports drink every 15 to 20 min. Most sports drinks in the 5%-10% carbohydrate concentration range are acceptable. However, some research suggests that a 6%-7% carbohydrate concentration range is better; studies have shown that a sports drink in this range is absorbed 30% faster than water and significantly faster than solutions exceeding 7% concentration.

Remember that cold liquids absorb into your system more rapidly. A practical tip is to freeze your sports drink in a water bottle before a long event. When you're ready to drink, it should be thawed out but still cold. Some helpful products include water bottles, water bottle covers, and water belts specifically designed to keep liquids cool.

Experiment to find the right drink for you, then plan your workouts and races accordingly. For races, find out what sports drink will be on the course and how far apart the aid stations will be. If it won't be your drink or if your pace won't get you to the aid stations within 15 min of each other, arrange to carry your fluids. On the run leg, this may mean using a water bottle holder or fluid-holding belt. The inconvenience will be well worth it.

Finally, feel free to use combinations of water, carbohydrate replacement drinks, and solid food, but any combinations should be tried and tested under similar training conditions before using them on race day.

Proper hydration during shorter events is clearly vital. Regardless of which sports drink you choose, the research points to the value of carbohydrate supplementation for longer endurance events, and some studies have shown moderate value for shorter, high-intensity training.

COFFEE ANYONE?

The International Olympic Committee defines caffeine in excess of 12 micrograms per millimeter of urine as a doping infraction. This is the equivalent of drinking 5 to 6 cups of coffee in a 2-hr period, something most people would have a hard time doing anyway.

As an ergogenic aid for athletes, caffeine spares muscle glycogen reserves by increasing metabolism and facilitating neuromuscular function. Some studies have shown that caffeine stimulates the central nervous system, thus limiting an athlete's perception of fatigue.

Many competitors swear by the strategy of ingesting caffeine before a race (within IOC limits), but there are many more who don't do well using caffeine. Caffeine can cause jitters and nervousness that may hinder performance. That cup of coffee also elevates your blood pressure and increases your heart rate. Caffeine is a diuretic, so any performance benefits may be negated by a mid-race pit stop at the porta-potty. Used in excess, caffeine can also cause dehydration and may increase lactic acid levels.

So when you look at the benefits versus the negative side effects, a cup of coffee before a race may not be such a good idea.

EATING FOR IMMUNITY

If you've ever run a marathon, you may feel a certain amount of irony that you've paid a race fee in return for (a) a few days of walking as though you're wearing diapers due to muscle soreness, (b) losing your ability to walk down stairs due to muscle tightness, (c) catching a cold or flu due to a weakened immune system.

Although postmarathon soreness and stiffness may be unavoidable, getting sick after a long competitive event or workout is a result of your body's vulnerability to infection—and it *isn't* inevitable. Your immune system just needs a boost.

The key to fortifying your immune system is balance—a balanced diet, balanced training. Research shows that moderate workouts, three times a week, strengthen the body against disease, but high-intensity training for longer periods of time may weaken the immune system. To prevent this effect, follow a balanced training program, take regular rest days, and maintain an adequate diet. If you feel a cold or flu coming on, modify your training schedule and incorporate more rest days and days off, depending on the severity of the symptoms.

Perhaps the best way to avoid these common ailments is to fortify the immune system through nutrition. Much scientific data suggests a link between building a fortresslike immune system and eating a balanced diet. Researchers have found that nutrients such as beta carotene, zinc, and vitamins E and C are essential to ward off the effects of "free radicals," which undermine our immunity to infection. The production of free radicals is also linked to strenuous exercise, so the extremely active woman has an increased likelihood of falling ill.

To maximize your body's resistance, you must balance more than 50 crucial nutrients, quite a balancing act. "What's good for the immune system is a balanced diet," says nutrition research specialist Dr. Jay Kenney, PhD, of the Pritikin Longevity Center in Santa Monica, California. "Research has shown us that a low-fat, high-carbohydrate diet strengthens the immune system, and a high-fat diet seems to suppress it."

You can put the odds in your favor by eating foods that contain considerable concentrations of these nutrients. Foods high in vitamin C include oranges, grapefruit, green peppers, strawberries, and cantaloupe. Foods high in beta carotene include carrots, sweet potatoes, dried apricots, and peaches. Vegetable oils and sunflower seeds contain vitamin E, but a low-fat source is wheat germ. As a general rule, most whole foods contain high concentrations of disease-preventive and immune-boosting compounds.

WHAT ABOUT BOOSTING IMMUNITY WITH SUPPLEMENTS?

Eating a balanced diet is great in theory, but actually doing it in our high-stress society of fast and processed foods can seem as difficult as running a sub-4-min mile.

Some research indicates that supplements can be beneficial in safeguarding the body against deficiencies of vital nutrients, but moderation is the key. Taken in excessive doses, vitamin C can hinder the absorption of copper. In addition, zinc supplements of more than 200 mg a day taken over an extended time can approach toxic levels.

Your best bet is a multivitamin and mineral supplement containing moderate amounts of vitamin C, vitamin E, zinc, and beta carotene.

LIVE FOOD, LIVE ENERGY

In recent years I have developed a personal interest in the benefits of eating "live food." You may cringe at the images that go through your mind, but the term *live food* doesn't refer to something that's still moving on your plate. Live food is anything organic that hasn't been processed, cooked, or had something done to it that has killed the live enzymes.

I learned that much of the food I ate regularly was "dead," and therefore, I was depleting my body's enzyme system. When the enzymes aren't present in the foods you eat, your body must draw on enzymes from your liver, pancreas, and other organs to break down and digest food, depleting their normal supply.

I realized that if I wanted to remedy the situation, I had a problem: I hated salads and raw vegetables. At the urging of a friend, I visited a local juice bar and tried a glass of carrot-apple juice with a dash of lime. I was astounded at how tasty this "live" drink was. I returned the next day and every day for the following 2 weeks. My energy levels began to increase, and the typical lulls during the afternoon and evening hours disappeared.

Now I own my own juicer. (The daily juice bar trips were getting to be very expensive.) I've even integrated wheat grass shots into my daily diet, which I call my "glasses of enzymes."

In our fast-paced society, eating dead food is the norm. But as athletes, it's in our best interest to concentrate on foods that help meet our unique nutritional needs, including our greater need for enzymes.

If you have an aversion to salads and raw vegetables, try a juicer. Like me, you'll probably be "juiced" for life.

THE FOOD GUIDE PYRAMID

The United States Department of Agriculture designed the Food Guide Pyramid as a guide to a healthy diet, based on its Dietary Guidelines. It's not a rigid prescription, but a general guide that can help you make healthy nutrition choices daily. The Pyramid calls for eating a variety of foods to get the nutrients you need and the right amount of calories to maintain healthy weight.

The Pyramid emphasizes foods from the five major food groups shown in three sections. At the base and second levels of the Pyramid are plenty of breads, cereals, rice, pasta, vegetables, and fruit, foods rich in carbohydrate. The milk and meat groups add moderate amounts of protein to your diet; nutrition authorities recommend low-fat dairy products and lean cuts of meat. Remember to go easy on fats, oils, and sweets, the foods at the tip of the Pyramid.

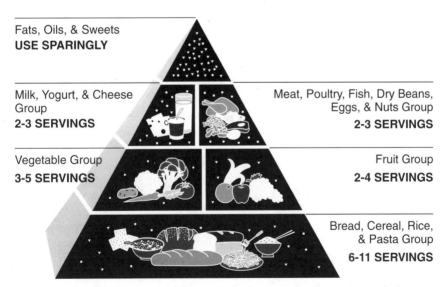

Fats, Oils, & Sweets
USE SPARINGLY

Milk, Yogurt, & Cheese Group
2-3 SERVINGS

Meat, Poultry, Fish, Dry Beans, Eggs, & Nuts Group
2-3 SERVINGS

Vegetable Group
3-5 SERVINGS

Fruit Group
2-4 SERVINGS

Bread, Cereal, Rice, & Pasta Group
6-11 SERVINGS

The USDA Food Guide Pyramid illustrates the importance of complex carbohydrates in your diet. Although the Pyramid was designed for the general public, athletes would do well to follow the general guidelines with a few modifications.

The Pyramid and You

While a diet that emphasizes carbohydrate is old news to endurance athletes, the USDA created the Food Guide Pyramid for the mainstream public. Although anyone can benefit from emphasis on carbohydrate, the Pyramid does not address the unique nutritional requirements of active women. Here are some important modifications you might want to consider:

- The active woman requires many more calories than the recommended servings contain. Modify by snacking on foods high in carbohydrate and low in fat between and with meals.

- For the female athlete burning a substantial amount of calories in training, increase the number of servings on the first and second levels of the Pyramid.

- Each serving recommended by the USDA is somewhat low in calories, ranging from 250 to 375. Another way to get the calories you need is to increase the serving size.

- Athletes need to be especially concerned about replenishing glycogen stores during long or intense training or competition. Sports drinks can be helpful in these situations.

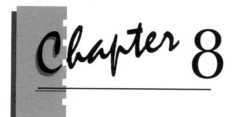

Chapter 8

Your Peak Fitness Workout Schedule

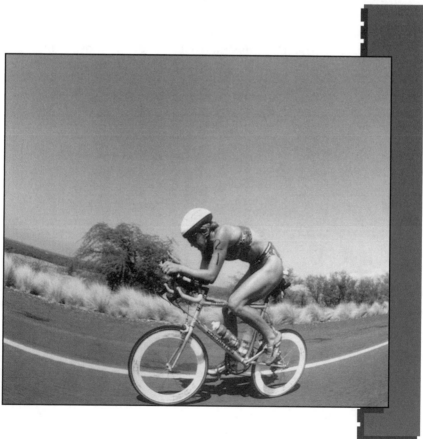

©Rich Cruse/RC Photo

157

We've spent a lot of time covering the components, guidelines, principles, and mechanics of peak fitness; I hope you have found the discussion helpful and applicable to your unique fitness goals. The next step is to show you how to apply what you've learned. You need a workable plan—a training schedule that will incorporate the three components of the Peak Fitness Triangle.

A TRAINING PROGRAM FOR YOU

Throughout this chapter, it's vital to keep in mind the need for individualizing the following information to fit your specific sport or exercise, as well as your unique goals.

Devising a training schedule can be a daunting, frustrating experience if you don't have any guidelines. Add to this the anxiety of recurring questions of diet, equipment choices, and the optimum race schedule and things can get pretty complicated.

It took many years for me to become comfortable with my training program, years of making adjustments and integrating new ideas that applied to me and my training goals. Part of the fun of training is finding new and different ways to adjust to life's challenges while continuing to make yourself more fit. However, with experience and knowledge, you should be able to train comfortably for an extended period with a program that you've individualized and that has had proven results.

Rest assured, if you can create a training schedule that works for *you*, and it's based on sound, scientific, common sense principles, then you'll be way ahead of the pack.

SETTING UP YOUR SCHEDULE

When setting up a training schedule, here are a few guidelines to keep in mind.

BE SENSIBLE ABOUT YOUR TIME

A common mistake when creating a training schedule is overestimating the time available to you during a normal day. Overestimating time to train can lead to feeling rushed and frustrated, which will turn your workouts into a chore rather than something you enjoy doing.

SET REALISTIC GOALS

Always remember to take your training one step at a time. Taking the long-term approach to training is even more crucial if you are just beginning to train in a new sport or partaking in a new form of physical activity.

THINK BALANCE

Don't sacrifice your family or your career for your fitness goals. Always keep in mind the priorities in your life. Unless you're a professional athlete, you shouldn't be working out all day. If you stick to your priorities and keep first things first, balance usually comes automatically. Still, if you find that your life is out of whack, maybe you're devoting too much time to training.

BE FLEXIBLE

A training program should be a user-friendly guide and a practical tool for attaining peak fitness. Don't be so rigid in executing your training that you sacrifice your health. Review the first section in chapter 7 and learn to understand the difference between natural muscle soreness and the soreness due to minor injury. Learn to tell the difference between being lazy and being overtrained. Be flexible, and adjust your schedule when your body needs rest.

PERIODIZE YOUR SCHEDULE

Set up a schedule that changes three or four times a year, according to what you want to accomplish within a 3- to 4-month period. Changing your schedule a few times a year makes sense and helps keep your mind fresh and your body challenged.

ALTERNATE INTENSITY

Understand the necessity of alternating the intensity of each session. A good schedule apportions a few days each week to work at a higher heart rate, while setting aside other days for lower intensity sessions. This is important if you want to improve in any chosen activity. Working at the same intensity day after day, week after week, will only ensure that you remain at the same fitness level or, more likely, slide backward.

SEEK EXPERT ADVICE

Don't be afraid to seek input from more experienced athletes about your training schedule. Talk to coaches to get their professional advice on setting up your program. Ultimately, however, you must take responsibility for finding whatever works best for you.

FEEL FREE TO BUCK THE TREND

If you find that something based on someone else's advice doesn't work, don't do it. Period.

WHAT CAN A COACH DO FOR YOU?

To achieve my peak performance, I consistently draw from a variety of experts in specialized fields related to sports and fitness. If you're serious about performance, someday you may want to consider seeking outside help, perhaps working with a coach.

You might be saying to yourself: *Why should I work with a coach? Who knows better than me how I should train?* Well, the acid test is competition—if you're consistently falling short of your goals, maybe you need outside help. It's hard to coach yourself because you don't have an objective view. A coach can help you see when you need to push harder as well as when you need a day off.

Participating in a coaching program can be a good way to learn the fundamentals of your sport. It's also a good idea to seek the advice of a coach when you decide to go for performance improvements, particularly speed. Any time you introduce speed into your training, it can open the door to injuries if not done properly. With coaching you'll learn to get faster safely.

If you find it difficult to devise a training schedule and aren't getting the results you want, good coaches can help you train under a structure that is safe, yet effective. They can help avoid such common training errors as undertraining, overtraining, and executing bad form. And good coaches will help you to train yourself better when they're not around.

How do you go about finding a coach? Your best bet is to ask other athletes with similar training and racing goals if they use a coach. Another alternative is to contact the local organization for your sport. To ensure that you find the skills you're looking for, I also suggest that you talk with a prospective coach and ask to sit in on a session or to participate in a trial workout.

TRAINING SCHEDULE COMPONENTS

Before we get into the training schedules, it's necessary to go over some of the terms and methods that are an integral part of this program.

KEY WORKOUTS

We talked about the key workout earlier, but I can't emphasize the value of these sessions enough. They should be the core of your training schedule. In most phases of my training program, key workouts are limited to one or two a week in each sport. (I sometimes go beyond that if I feel I need to and that my body can handle it safely.) These sessions are the foundations of my training, and they rarely change in structure. They are my "bread-and-butter" work. During these workouts, I focus all my energy—mentally, physically, emotionally—in every possible way.

Key workouts are the best measure of my peak fitness and are the acid tests for speed, endurance, and strength. After a key workout, I can accurately judge where I am on my own performance scale. Key workouts are a much better measure of fitness than total mileage because, even though you're racking up the miles, weaknesses such as lack of speed, endurance, or strength may be camouflaged.

For most of the year, the group workouts I attend—the Monday Carlsbad Swim, the Tuesday Run, and the Wednesday Ride I described in chapter 2—are my key workouts.

PACE

Three terms are used to designate the ideal pace for a workout. Below is a brief description of each, with examples from my training and racing workouts.

Easy

This is the slowest possible pace. If your maximum heart rate is 180, these workouts should be executed at about 120 to 130. Give yourself the talk test: you should be able to hold a conversation during these workouts without difficulty. An easy run for me is about an 8-min pace.

Steady

A steady pace is similar to the speed at which I would be doing an Ironman-distance race, which is about 160 beats/min. On a steady run, I'll be at a 7-min pace.

Hard

This is threshold work, at about 170 beats/min for me. On a run, I will be at a sub-6-min pace. On a bicycle, I may be averaging 25 mph.

TIME AND DISTANCE

You'll notice that on the upcoming training schedules, I use time and distance interchangeably. That's because for some workouts, I focus on distance, and for others, I'm more concerned with being out there a certain amount of time. It's simply my preference. It probably doesn't matter much whether you choose to structure your sessions by time or by distance (although if you're going to choose one, I'd suggest you focus on time rather than become obsessed with mileage).

DOUBLE WORKOUTS

You'll also note that on some days I do two workouts in one sport. If you can commit to that level of training, doing double workouts is a feasible way to get the most out of your day. If your first session is hard or long, a second round later in the day might help your body flush out lactic acid. To allow your muscles enough time to recover, always schedule the sessions as far apart as possible, preferably one in the early morning and the other in the evening. In between, make sure you eat right, stretch, and if possible, get a massage.

AM/PM

Where appropriate, I've also noted the time of day of training with either an "AM" or a "PM" designation. I've done this to help you see how I space out more than one session in a day to give my body enough rest. Usually the PM workouts are easy and are designed to loosen me up and avoid muscular tightness.

PERIODIZATION

My program is based on periodization, with the Gatorade® Ironman World Championship Triathlon in the fall being the one event my entire year is focused on. You may want to focus on a particular race, or perhaps your goal is noncompetitive. In any case, you can still use the concept of periodization and modify accordingly, as we'll discuss in greater detail later.

INTERVAL TRAINING

A component of the following schedules that deserves special consideration is interval training, sometimes referred to as speed work. Most of my key workouts are structured around the concept of interval training. For the serious athlete, interval training is a key element in improving speed. Although interval training differs from sport to sport, here are some basic guidelines to follow.

Establish Your Base

A cautionary note is warranted with any kind of speed work—you should have a solid base of long-distance training. Intervals require greater muscle strength and impose higher cardiovascular and respiratory demands. Translation: intervals are hard work and can easily cause injuries unless you're in decent shape.

Decide What You Want

Focus your interval training on a performance goal at a specific race. If you're not training for competition, it's helpful to have a tangible goal, so base your interval workouts on a specific measure of performance.

Plan Your Other Workouts Accordingly

Do your interval workouts once a week and try to position them on a day that isn't too close to other hard workouts. For example, if you're a runner and do a hard track workout on Friday that leaves your legs feeling like spaghetti, Saturday would not be a good day to participate in a hard group run.

Allow yourself an easy day, both before and after your speed workout. If you don't, you're risking injury. Also, don't do a speed workout in the week preceding a race (if you expect to finish before the volunteers go home).

Choose the Appropriate Distance

Interval workouts will be different for someone who is training for a short-distance race than for someone who is training for a long event. The longer the distance you are training for, the longer your interval distance should be, although the number of intervals will be fewer.

For example, if you're training for a long-distance running race, you should be running either 1/2-mi or 1-mi intervals (or a combination of both). A typical marathon workout might be six 1/2-mi intervals or four 1-mi repeats. For shorter races, your workout should consist of a combination of 1/2-mi and 1/4-mi repeats (although it wouldn't be a bad idea to throw in some 1-mi intervals once in awhile).

Start Small and Work Your Way Up

The first time you do an interval workout, do two repeats of any distance you choose and increase it by two each week. Do this until you're totaling middle-distance mileage (not including warm-ups, cooldowns, or recoveries).

Go for Consistency

The most common mistake athletes make when tackling intervals is blowing up after the first few. The goals are consistency and getting your body to adapt to prolonged hard efforts (as in a race). You're not going to teach your body—and your mind—good pace-setting skills by having erratic interval times.

Use your watch and record your times after each repeat. If there is more than a 5-s difference in your repeats, you need to fine-tune your internal pace clock. If you have a watch that beeps, set it for your interval goal. Focus on that time and try to finish exactly when you hear the beep. It may take a few attempts, but you'd be surprised at how exact your body can be at matching a pace to your internal clock.

Concentrate on Form

A major benefit of speed work is that it improves your form. It teaches your body to focus on biomechanical improvements and to exercise efficiently. Keep this in mind when doing your intervals, and concentrate on smooth execution. There's no greater experience during a running track workout, for example, than to feel like you're a flying, smooth-running gazelle.

Make It Fun

Interval workouts can be fun. (Okay, you can laugh, but I'm being semiserious here.) For example, many group workouts are rewarding social experiences. The drawback is that you won't get a workout specific to your training goal, but you can always duck out if it's too long or stay longer if it's too short.

Vary your workouts, too; don't do the same workout every week. If you're running, cycling, or in-line skating and have a measured, more scenic course, feel free to do your workout there. If you don't overdo it, you'll soon be relishing the feeling of gliding along the track, path, or road—and reveling in smashing all your previous race records.

THE PEAK FITNESS TRAINING SCHEDULE

When I did my first triathlon in 1985, while still living in South Africa, my only resources in putting together a program were triathlon training books by Dave Scott and Scott Tinley. When I studied the chapters that outlined their training schedules, I was mortified. I didn't have the time or the inclination to put in all the mileage they recommended.

I made the mistake of chucking the whole idea of putting together a schedule. I just followed the pack, training the way everyone around me trained. When I woke up in the morning, I was never sure what I would be doing, much less why I was doing it. As a result, my athletic performances were very inconsistent. Sometimes I would have a great race, only to find myself slipping the week after.

Years later, when I moved to Southern California, I began taking note of the schedules of the top athletes around me, particularly those who seemed to have a specific purpose for each training session and who had consistent success on the race circuit. Based on these observations, I began a process of "individualization," adapting these training techniques to my specific goals and circumstances.

I recommend that you take the same approach to the information presented here. Each person has different training goals and time commitments, so rather than attempting to accommodate every scheduling possibility, I've outlined my weekly training schedule in the next few pages.

In addition, my training is triathlon-specific. If you participate in other sports, such as in-line skating, mountain biking, or cross-country skiing, you will need to modify the schedule by relating to the *types* of workouts shown here. In this case, it will be more useful to look at the *purpose* of each phase and the *structure* of each schedule rather than the content.

Following this section, I'll discuss how you can use my training program as a template and modify it to create your own path to peak fitness.

THE BASE TRAINING PHASE

I see my base training as a "breaking-in" period when I'm preparing my body for the rigors of the intensity and longer training of upcoming phases. Emphasis is on building strength and endurance, step by step and little by little.

Duration

I start base training at the beginning of the calendar year, although I've maintained some sort of alternative (fun) exercise program, such as mountain biking or in-line skating, in the prior months. This phase usually lasts about 5 months, so I begin the next phase of training in June.

Key Workouts

The goal of key workouts is to develop an endurance base. Thus the emphasis is on longer workouts for cardiovascular conditioning, although I may start to focus on speed toward the latter part of this phase to prepare me for the next stage.

Strength Training

Here's how I integrate the peak fitness strength training program with my base training phase:

1. For the first 3 weeks during the base training phase, I work with the acclimation phase, which is most of January for me.

2. Then I work with the strength and endurance phase for 5 weeks, until the end of February.

3. Beginning in March, I work for 4 weeks on the power and endurance phase.

4. Throughout April and May, I work with the peak power phase and then transition to the maintenance phase.

Flexibility

The frequency and structure of flexibility training remains a constant throughout these phases.

Things to Remember

- Always increase your mileage safely. Use the "10% rule" of increasing your mileage no more than 10% each week. And every other week, decrease your total mileage to give your body some recovery time.

- Don't feel as though you're not working hard enough if you aren't going all out with each workout. Base training means a lot of long, slow distance work designed to get the body accustomed to the biomechanics of your exercise and to the rigors of endurance. Be patient with yourself until you're ready for speed training.

Base Training Key Workouts

Table 8.1 outlines your base training schedule.

Monday's swim: This workout is part of my swimming group session, the Carlsbad Masters Swim Program. After a brief warm-up, my main set is six to eight 400-m repeats at race pace, with 20 to 30 s of rest.

Tuesday's run: The morning run is the Tuesday Run. It is a 12-mi group run on a partly hilly trail, combined with intervals on a flat golf course, and ending with a very long, steep hill. This run helps me to develop speed, strength, and endurance, although early on I stick with a slower group of runners and concentrate on the latter. Even if you decide not to join a group, find a course that offers all the challenges of this one; it will not only help you develop running strength and stamina, but more important, it will teach you how to pace yourself.

Wednesday's ride: The Wednesday Ride is an essential component of my cycling training. The pace is easy and steady the first half, then hard, fast, and furious on the way back.

Table 8.1   The Base Training Schedule

| Day | Cardiovascular Conditioning | | | Strength | Flexibility |
	Swimming	Cycling	Running	Weights	Stretching
Mon.	**3,200 m**	1.5-2 hr	5-6 mi		Pilates stretch class (90 min)
Tue.	1,500 m, easy		**AM: 12 mi, hard, hilly run** PM: 4mi, easy	AM: weights	
Wed.	3,000 m	**70-mi group ride**	PM: 7 mi, easy		
Thu.	1,500 m, easy		1 hr, steady, hill run	AM: weights	PM: 45 min
Fri.	3,000 m, intervals	2 hr, easy	PM: 45 min, easy		
Sat.		**4-5 hr, steady**	PM: 30 min, easy		
Sun.	1,500 m, easy		**1.5 hr, steady**	PM: weights	45 min after weights

Note: Key workouts are in bold.

Adapted from *The Total Triathlon Almanac*, copyright 1993 by Tony Svensson. The almanac is a combined training log and fitness handbook used by endurance athletes. Published by Trimarket, Palo Alto, CA.

Saturday's ride: If I can, I try to make this a hilly mountain bike ride early in the morning and then relax most of the rest of the day. I manage to get in an easy jog in the afternoon to work the kinks (lactic acid) out of my legs. Toward the end of the base training phase, my Saturday rides are closer to 6 hr.

Sunday's run: This is a steady-paced hill run that is about 13 mi long, although I concentrate on the quality of the workout time rather than on distance. Toward the end of this phase, my runs last as long as 2 hr.

THE SPEED TRAINING PHASE

The transition from base strength and endurance to power and speed occurs in this phase. Thus, each key workout is structured and executed at a faster pace, and the mileage is significantly reduced.

Duration

This phase can last 4 months, from June until September on my training calendar.

Key Workouts

As with all the workouts, the key workouts are reduced in mileage. I limit myself to one key workout per discipline and focus on speed and performance. I also do some racing on weekends.

Strength Training

During this training phase, my sessions are a shortened version of off-season or winter strength training. Because of time limitations and the pressures of racing during this period, I usually cut the time I spend in the weight room to a bare minimum. Weight training is integrated in the following manner:

1. I start racing late in May, so I don't do any weights again until mid-July.
2. Starting in mid-July, I spend 2 weeks on the acclimation phase.
3. Starting the beginning of August, I spend 3 weeks in the strength and endurance phase.
4. From the last week of August until early or mid-September, I work on the power and endurance phase.

Flexibility

You'll see from the schedules that I find it helpful to stretch after weight training or running. Because your body is warmed up, the gains in range of motion from stretching after these activities can be significant.

Things to Remember

- In this phase, you're most likely to overtrain and perhaps feel mentally burned out. (I remedy that situation by traveling and training in Boulder for a month or two in July or August. Not only is the altitude training beneficial, but the change of scenery, training partners, and terrain gives me a fresh perspective.) You may not be able to get away for a month, but even a weekend getaway or change in terrain can be helpful.

- When working out in a group, don't fall into the trap of staying with people who are faster than you. The idea is for others to push you, but not so far beyond your current fitness level that you're limping home.

- You may choose not to race during this phase and concentrate on interval and high-intensity work. The following chart is for training during the week of a Sunday race. Instead of a race, substitute a workout that would somewhat simulate the conditions of a race. (For me, that usually means a hilly and hard 45-min ride followed immediately by a 5-mi run.)

Speed Training Key Workouts

Table 8.2 outlines your speed training schedule.

Monday's swim: No change, although I definitely try to maintain a race pace for each interval.

Tuesday's run: If I participate in the group run, I complete it in a faster time, usually 12 mi under 1:10. Otherwise I stick to short intervals on a track to peak my running speed and optimize my form. My track sessions usually consist of 10 to 12 400-m intervals at faster than race pace, approximately 90% of maximum heart rate. But don't start with 10 intervals if you haven't been doing track work; begin with 2 and work your way up safely.

Wednesday's ride: Naturally, the higher level of fitness seems to spawn a flurry of competition, and the group rides tend to be severe and fast, which is physically and mentally draining (although they are a little shorter). I try to stick with the faster groups, especially the faster men, if I can.

Table 8.2 The Speed Training Schedule

Day	Cardiovascular Conditioning			Strength	Flexibility
	Swimming	Cycling	Running	Weights	Stretching
Mon.	**3,200 m**	1.5-2 hr	5-6 mi		45 min after running
Tue.	1,500 m, easy		**AM: high intensity, short intervals** PM: 30 min, easy	PM: weights (see details above)	
Wed.	3,000 m	**45-50 mi, hard**	PM: 7 mi, easy		
Thu.	1,500 m, easy		AM: 1 hr, steady, hill run	PM: weights	PM: 45 min after weights
Fri.			30 min, easy		
Sat.	800 m, easy (optional)	30 min, easy	30 min, easy		PM: 30 min, light session
Sun.	Race/similar high-intensity workout				

Note: Key workouts are in bold.

Adapted from *The Total Triathlon Almanac*, copyright 1993 by Tony Svensson. The almanac is a combined training log and fitness handbook used by endurance athletes. Published by Trimarket, Palo Alto, CA.

THE PEAK TRAINING PHASE

By the end of the speed training phase, you should be at a high level of fitness. The peak training phase is a very short phase designed to focus on the specific event or competition. Peak training is high-intensity physical and mental training that is totally centered on a single target: a race or goal.

Duration

This phase lasts just 3 weeks, although you may prefer to make it as long as 6 weeks. However, don't spend too much time in this phase; it's very exhausting, both physically and mentally. You should always feel like you've peaked your body for your target, not like you have nothing left to give when you're on the starting line.

Key Workouts

I focus on giving 110% during the key workouts in each sport. I am also more mentally focused each session, using visualization techniques during my training frequently.

Strength Training

I choose not to do any weight training during this phase; I've done my homework in the weight room, and the work I've done thus far has significantly increased my strength. My main focus is on cardio-vascular conditioning. Instead of weight training, I find it helpful and relaxing to substitute surgical tubing (stretch cord) exercises after my runs.

Flexibility

Devote a little more time to stretching during this phase; however, because of the level of fatigue your muscles and joints will be experiencing, be careful not to hurt yourself.

Things to Remember

- On the surface, the peak training phase may appear to be somewhat identical to the base training phase. It's more a matter of approach than content. Your pace should be significantly increased, and you should be giving each key workout your total concentration and effort. You should be using some of the mental techniques described in chapter 6.

- Because of the intensity of this stage, you are susceptible to injury here as well. Take note of any pain around the joints or any of the other overtraining signals described in chapter 7.

- In this phase, little things matter a great deal, so focus on nutrition, massage, stretching, and other activities that are good for your body.

Peak Training Key Workouts

Table 8.3 outlines your peak training schedule.

Monday's swim: Same workout, although the distance is slightly longer. After warm-up, I usually do 8 to 10 400-m intervals at an Ironman pace.

Tuesday's run: Same workouts, although I make a special effort to go hard and finish with a good time.

Wednesday's ride: Hammering hard as usual.

Friday's ride: This ride is very race-specific for me. I ride for 4 to 5 hr at an Ironman pace, staying very focused on a course where I know there will be few stops. I try to simulate race conditions, even down to the fluids I will be drinking and the foods I will be eating during the Ironman.

Friday's run: I do this as soon as I get off the bike, although I start slowly and eat foods that I will eat during the race. I stay focused on my running rhythm and on setting a steady pace. This workout is designed more for "feeling" than for speed.

Saturday's run: Another race-specific workout. If my goal is a 3-hr marathon in the Ironman, I run at a 7-min pace or faster. My legs are usually fatigued from Friday's long ride, which makes for an ideal simulation of the Ironman. Again, any fluids or solids are the same ones I may ingest during the race. Note: I always do this run alone so I can concentrate totally on pacing myself. You may want to do the same.

MODIFYING YOUR TRAINING SCHEDULE

Although this program is time-consuming, it is designed for optimum fitness and peak performance in an ultradistance triathlon event.

Table 8.3   The Peak Training Schedule

| Day | Cardiovascular Conditioning | | | Strength | Flexibility |
	Swimming	Cycling	Running	Weights	Stretching
Mon.	**4,000 m**	1.5 hr, easy	5-6 mi, easy		PM: 45 min
Tue.	1,500 m, easy	1.5 hr, moderate	**AM: 12 mi, hard, hilly run** PM: 5 mi, easy (optional)	PM: surgical tubing exercises after second run	
Wed.	3,000 m	**70-mi group ride**	PM: 6-8 mi, easy		
Thu.	1,500 m, easy		AM: 1 hr, steady, hill run PM: 4-5 mi, easy	PM: surgical tubing exercises after second run	PM: 45 min
Fri.	1,000 m, easy ocean swim	**90 mi, steady**	**5 mi, steady**		
Sat.			**2-2.5 hr, steady**		
Sun.	1,500 m, easy		1 hr, very slow		45 min after run

Note: Key workouts are in bold.

Adapted from *The Total Triathlon Almanac*, copyright 1993 by Tony Svensson. The almanac is a combined training log and fitness handbook used by endurance athletes. Published by Trimarket, Palo Alto, CA.

Use the preceding schedules as a template and the periodization structure as a general guideline for accomplishing your unique goal. Below are some additional principles that I've used to construct my training schedule; you can use them to modify your own program.

- Vary the distances or lengths of your training sessions.
- Integrate the three components of the Peak Fitness Triangle into your schedule: cardiovascular conditioning, strength, and flexibility.
- Always start with base training first, then move on to more specific training, whether this means more distance or more speed.
- Try to do at least one workout a week in a group environment, preferably one in each discipline. Group workouts provide structure as well as simulating some of the pressures of competition, which will help you to push harder (if you want to keep up). And they're fun too.
- Whether you're competitive or not, schedule some off-season time doing activities that are not part of your regular regimen. If you just can't break away from your sport for any length of time, at least vary the terrain, environment, distance, pace, or any number or combination of variables. You may not believe you need it, but giving your body and mind some variety pays off in the long run.

MIDDLE- AND SHORT-DISTANCE TRIATHLON TRAINING MODIFICATIONS

If your goal is a medium- or short-distance event, such as an Olympic-distance or sprint triathlon, the first thing you need to modify is the distance or duration of each training session. The preceding schedule is easily adaptable by modifying the key workouts to be event-specific and scaling down the mileage for the rest of your training. Examples of key workouts for middle- and short-distance triathlon goals appear in Table 8.4.

CREATING YOUR OWN SCHEDULE

Now it's time to sit down and do some homework. Use the blank templates in Tables 8.5 through 8.7 to create your peak fitness training schedule for each phase of the year.

Table 8.4   Middle- and Short-Distance Key Workout Examples

	Olympic-Distance Triathlon	Sprint-Distance Triathlon
Swim	Four 6 × 400-m intervals	8 × 200-m intervals
Ride	40-60 mi steady riding, with a few sprints and climbs	30 mi with a 10- to 15-mi time trial at race pace or faster
Run	8- to 9-mi fartlek run (Throw in five or six hard surges throughout the middle of your run.)	Track workout: 8 x 400-m intervals at faster than race pace

KEEPING A TRAINING LOG

No matter what sport(s) you participate in, an essential element of your training program should be maintaining an accurate log of your daily and weekly workouts. A diary that chronicles the variables that affect your energy level and performance can help you achieve peak fitness.

The fun of keeping a log or journal is that you can record thoughts and feelings about your training and racing—comments and notes you can later associate with joy (or regret).

On a practical level, a more detailed training log can be a tool for objectively monitoring your progress. In addition, you can use it to spot trends and avoid patterns that lead to injury. Depending on how detailed you choose to make your log, it can become your personal database, with access to volumes of information just a page flip away.

Ultimately, the type of log you maintain depends on your personality. Whereas a detailed, highly specific log that includes numerous metrics may appeal to the organized and logical, a more casual journal or diary that records little more than workouts, feelings, and other observations may appeal to a different type.

Whether you opt to keep a highly detailed training log that resembles the command console of the *Starship Enterprise,* or something much simpler, what's most important is that you keep it updated consistently. Establish a set time to write, whether it's immediately after a workout when your senses are still reeling from the effort, or after a cool shower when you've had time to think.

Table 8.5 Your Base Training Schedule   Start Date: End Date:

Day	Cardiovascular Conditioning			Strength Weights			Flexibility Stretching
Mon.							
Tue.							
Wed.							
Thu.							
Fri.							
Sat.							
Sun.							

Note: Circle or underline key workouts.

Table 8.6   Your Speed Training Schedule

Start Date: _____   End Date: _____

Day	Cardiovascular Conditioning		Strength Weights	Flexibility Stretching
Mon.				
Tue.				
Wed.				
Thu.				
Fri.				
Sat.				
Sun.				

Note: Circle or underline key workouts.

Table 8.7 Your Peak Training Schedule   **Start Date:**   **End Date:**

Day	Cardiovascular Conditioning			Strength Weights		Flexibility Stretching	
Mon.							
Tue.							
Wed.							
Thu.							
Fri.							
Sat.							
Sun.							

Note: Circle or underline key workouts.

What are the benefits of keeping a log? Several of my colleagues keep a log, and each one gets something different out of it. Many say their logs give them clues to what caused an injury or a poor performance.

Professional triathlete Karen Smyers has kept a training log throughout her athletic career: "My training log is not really scientific, but it's tremendously helpful," she says. "I frequently go back and look at where I was last year, or pinpoint when I timed a particular type of workout. It gives me a good idea of how I'm doing now."

Although her log consists only of descriptions of each workout or race and any key results and comments on how she felt, it's enough to indicate to her whether she's allowing herself sufficient time to recover. It also helps her to establish what works and what doesn't work by analyzing patterns and trends.

"I remember a race a few years ago where I was at least three or four minutes slower than the previous week's race. When I went back to my journal, I saw that every workout during the week had been hard."

A log doesn't have to be a method of pinpointing errors in training. It can also be used as a tool to enhance performance. After an awe-inspiring performance, a look back at your log can help you determine some of the factors that led to that breakthrough, or possibly help you establish your optimum tapering schedule before competition.

COMPUTERIZED LOGS

If you own a computer, many software programs are available that can serve as your log. Most computer logs (such as the one on p. 181) give you the option of recording workouts in many different sports and usually include space for the categories described on pp. 182-183, as well as room for notes and comments about your workout.

One of the greatest advantages of a computer log is the graphics, which can tell you at a glance how your training is progressing (see p. 181).

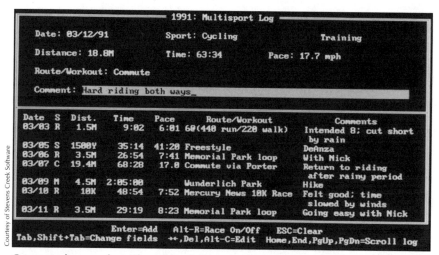

Computer logs, such as The Athlete's Diary, make keeping track of your workouts fun and easy.

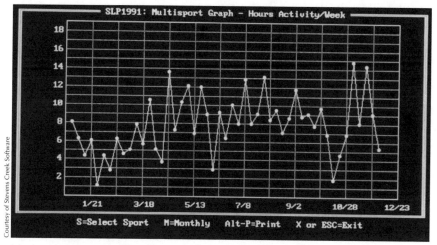

Most computer programs offer a graph mode that allows you to see the progress of your exercise program measured by time, pace, or distance.

CREATING YOUR INDIVIDUAL LOG

There are numerous preprinted training logs, but you can also create an individualized log with a spiral notebook and a ruler. For those who thrive on detail, here are some variables to make sure you include in your training log.

Hours Slept

Although current research suggests moderate sleep deprivation has little effect on performance during the adrenaline high of competition, normal training may be affected. So that ragged feeling during a 10-mi training jog may be the result of too little snooze time.

Waking Pulse

Record your beats per minute when you wake up, preferably while you're still in bed. An increase of more than 3 or 4 beats can signal overtraining. Although we discussed several overtraining signals in chapter 7, waking pulse is the best way to measure the need for rest. My resting pulse is between 38 and 40, so if I wake and find my pulse at 44 or higher, I'll make my workout easy or take the day off.

Distances

Tracking correct distances for measured sports can keep you honest. It is also the most obvious measurement for checking your progress.

Time of Day

Energy levels fluctuate during the day according to many factors that are unique to each individual. As long as all other variables remain the same, you can pinpoint your peak time of day for a workout.

Intensity

Describe the intensity of your workout or race. There are many ways to do this, but the more specific you are, the better. You could use a scale of 1 to 5, or use descriptions such as "easy," "slightly difficult," "moderate," "hard," "very hard," and "brutal." Monitoring intensity levels is the key to avoiding too many back-to-back killer workouts.

Mood

Although mood can be affected by many things, it is sometimes a precursor of illness and an indication of overtraining. For example, irritability is an early sign that you're pushing yourself too hard.

Injury Flags

Pay close attention to any unusual pain—especially around the joints, where most injuries occur.

Weight

Get on the scale in the morning, after you're relieved yourself. A 3% or greater loss of body weight may mean you've lost too much fluid. Make it an easy day, or better yet, take a day off.

Personal Notes

Perhaps the best part about keeping a training log is flipping back to read about that special workout, the one with the funny story, or that glimpse of Olympic potential. Babble on—you deserve it.

Chapter 9

Competing at
Your Best

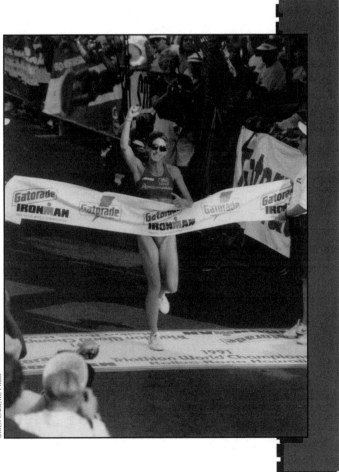

If you've ever watched the Gatorade® Ironman World Championship Triathlon in Hawaii on television, you've only caught a glimpse of the special web of magic this race weaves around everyone involved in it. If you want to experience human drama and touch the heart of what it means to be the best possible athlete, the best possible self you can be, go and watch.

Reserve a spot in the bleachers near the finish line on Alii Drive early in the morning, hours before the athletes begin running, limping, and sometimes crawling in. The seats will be gone by early afternoon, every last one of them, which is amazing considering that triathlon is not exactly a spectator sport. (Many consider watching a triathlon the equivalent of watching grass grow.) Unlike the summary coverage on television, with its great underwater action shots of the swim, the fast moves on the bike course, the heart-stopping surges on the run, and the dramatic soundtrack music throughout, watching a triathlon in person can be pretty boring much of the time.

Nevertheless, the bleacher seats in Kona are filled to capacity long before the winners arrive. And they continue to stay full, standing room only, in fact, until well after midnight, until the very last person crosses the finish line. The decibel level is unbelievable; waves of cheers from spectators can be heard a mile away on the run course, a welcome sound to the weary Ironman athlete.

Why the big crowd? Why all the fuss?

I suppose to a lot of people, the Gatorade® Ironman Triathlon is nothing but an event designed to produce profits, or to the media, simply a noteworthy event to report to the public. But to triathletes, it is the ultimate challenge. It is a place where the best, and a few lucky enough to get in by lottery, test their mettle, not only against each other but against searing heat, deafening crosswinds, and unfriendly terrain.

Simply put, it's one of the endurance world's biggest challenges—and a great place to discover or reaffirm *what makes people good.*

If you can't make it to Kona, go watch any marathon or triathlon. Try to get near the finish line, where I'm sure you'll also be hard-pressed to find a good seat or someplace to stand.

See for yourself.

THE MEANING OF COMPETITION

As a professional athlete, competition naturally has some serious connotations for me. When I "toe up" to the starting line on a beach, money, fame, honor, reputation, all of it is on the line. Yet, for the person committed to fitness, performing at peak fitness when it counts the most, in competition, is just as serious an endeavor.

The financial and professional considerations may not be there, but the personal and emotional rewards can be infinitely more gratifying—or just as elusive—as prize money.

I chose to end my book with the subject of competition because it is during a contest that everything we've discussed so far will come together. In the first half of this chapter, I'll relate many of my valuable personal experiences to give you some insight into how a rival can help you on your quest for peak performance. In the latter portion, I'll tell you some practical things you can do that will help you perform at your best.

ME AND MY SHADOW

Our first meeting was at the 1986 Ironman, but I'd heard of Erin Baker a year earlier. Clearly one of the world's best, she was unable to participate in America due to visa problems, but once her traveling woes had been settled, she promptly took the triathlon circuit by storm. Since then it has been all-out war between Erin and me, due in large part to the media.

In 1990, ABC aired the Ironman Triathlon to millions of viewers, showing pictures of us mimicking arm wrestling, glaring at each other, oiled muscles tensed, two warrior women locked in a piercing gaze. In the 1991 NBC broadcast, John Tesh again highlighted our rivalry with interviews from both of us—not about our thoughts on the race—but about each other.

To make the rivalry even more colorful, the media has always depicted us as total opposites. I've always been depicted as mild-mannered and quietly confident (the "good guy"), Erin as brash and arrogant (the "bad guy"). Good against evil. Luke Skywalker and Darth Vader. According to the media, our rivalry is the endurance world's version of *Star Wars*.

Even though all the media hype has made it seem as though we couldn't wait to get at each other's throats, the rivalry between myself and Erin Baker has helped lift me to many a peak performance. Webster's defines *rivalry* as "one of two striving to obtain something that only one can possess." That, in brief, defines my relationship with Erin Baker.

Because we are so equal in talent, because we are also—when you get right down to it—very much alike, we unnerve each other. She and I have the same mental toughness, the same fierce commitment to winning, the same focused concentration. Where other athletes will crumble when pain sets in, Erin, like me, will just bear down harder.

DEVELOPING A HEALTHY RIVALRY

Although my rivalry with Erin Baker occurred purely by chance, you can develop a rivalry to help you perform at your best during competition. There is a fundamental human need to be respected and recognized by your peers. When you compete against someone of equal or greater ability in a healthy, safe environment, such as a race or an organized event, it can lift your energy level and mental concentration to new heights.

Exactly how do you go about finding someone you'd like to demoralize, pummel to the ground, beat to a pulp? Wait a minute! First you must realize that healthy competition isn't hostile or negative. Instead of wishing a competitor ill fortune, the healthy athlete wants a rival to succeed so that they can both rise to a whole new level.

Among the professional triathlon community, even though we are all in direct competition with each other, many of us work out together and share new training concepts.

Most professional triathletes participate in some sort of group workout, whether it be the Tuesday Run, the Wednesday Ride, or the Masters Swim program in Carlsbad. Instead of hostility and antagonism, the pervading feelings at most group workouts are quite jovial, with underlying feelings of camaraderie. That's not to say that we don't compete against each other—the competition is fierce.

This is unheard of in the world of professional athletics, where oftentimes new training protocols are well-guarded, kept from the competition like top secret government documents. Most triathletes are willing to go out of their way to share new training techniques, whether it's a new exercise routine, a tapering program, or the latest piece of cycling equipment. This makes triathlon a sport ahead of its time.

It's easy to misunderstand my recommendation to focus on a rival as something negative, and I know many would say such an approach creates conflict and puts undue pressure on an athlete from external forces. We discussed how important it is to avoid comparisons and expectations in chapter 6, which may seem to run counter to developing any sort of rivalry. But there is an important distinction. Taken in the right context, *a healthy rivalry can help you to focus inward*. It can help you focus on your own best performance for a positive effect, if taken *in the context* of the competition around you.

Sports psychologists agree that too much stress can have a negative effect on performance, and in no way am I advocating introducing negative stress into training and racing. However, a certain degree of positive stress can be very beneficial and can motivate you to work harder. The key is to see your rivalry as your guiding light, as a tool you can use to find the potential within yourself.

Should your rival be your training partner? Most likely, your relationship with your rival won't have the negative connotations caused by all the media hype that has surrounded Erin and me. However, I would caution against training with your rival for a very important reason: the tendency to throw out your training schedule in the heat of battle. A common cause of injury is the inclination among highly competitive athletes to exceed the limits of a smart and safe training plan during a heated workout duel.

If you find yourself consistently overtraining and pushing yourself beyond your current capabilities under the pressure of training with your competition, you're better off limiting the battles to organized events.

If you have enough self-discipline to stay within your current fitness limitations, even during the heat of a duel, training with your rival may be beneficial. Still, you may want to limit your sessions with your "special" training partner to key workouts within your speed training or peak fitness phases. The intensity of these sessions will usually be higher, and your body will likely be more able to handle a pace increase.

Who can be a rival? A rival can be anyone, even your best friend or your spouse. (I've seen competitions between husband and wife get pretty intense.) It's not important who the person is, but rather that he or she motivate you—for whatever reason—to compete at your peak.

THE MECHANICS OF COMPETITION

Preparation is everything in athletics. It amazes me that so many outstanding athletes will spend months, sometimes years, preparing for a single event, only to ruin their chances by not following some simple—although subtle—commonsense strategies. The weeks and days preceding an important event should be planned and executed as meticulously as any other phase of training. So, let's look at some practical concerns every athlete should consider when preparing for competition.

TAPERING FOR PEAK PERFORMANCE

The value of tapering is something that endurance athletes have known for a long time. Nevertheless, I still hear stories of the competitor who insists on putting in one last hard workout the day before a race, only to find herself exhausted even before she toes up at the starting line.

As mentioned in the previous chapter, my peak training phase is 3 weeks of high-intensity, totally focused workouts. Then I begin to taper for the Gatorade® Ironman Triathlon, and when I taper, I take it pretty seriously. The goal of my tapering program is to end up on the beach in Kona feeling as though I could have done one more long workout. Too often, athletes find themselves physically and mentally exhausted at the starting line from months of hard training and no tapering plan.

Tapering consists of decreasing exercise intensity, volume, or a combination of both before a race. The subject of tapering inevitably spawns the key question: *How much, when, and will it do me any good?* A recent study reported in *Running Times*, conducted at Malaspina College in British Columbia and the University of Alberta, provides some answers. In the study, 25 athletes trained for 1 hr, 5 days a week, for 6 weeks at a high intensity level of 75% to 85% of $\dot{V}O_2$max.

After 6 weeks, seven athletes tapered for 3 days, cutting down on volume (not intensity), and a second group tapered for 6 days. A third group tapered by doing no exercise at all for 4 full days, and an unfortunate bunch in the fourth group exercised at the same intensity and volume until test day (equivalent to race day).

The results showed a 12% increase in the lactic acid threshold level in both the 3-day and 6-day taper groups. (The lactic acid threshold is a measure of how long a certain exercise intensity can be maintained.) The "no-exercise" group made no improvement, and the "train-to-death" group actually decreased their lactic threshold level. The level of carbohydrate stores (glycogen storage levels) soared by 25% with the 6-day program. The 3-day and the no-exercise groups showed an increase of 12%. Once again, the train-to-death group points to overtraining: their glycogen levels dropped 12%.

"My focus was the cellular level, finding the physiological results of tapering. Of course, everybody wants to know about performance," says J.P. Neary, PhD, who headed the study. "The results determine that a little extra rest helps cells work more efficiently during exercise."

Neary emphasizes that tapering is subject to a host of variables specific to the individual and the training event. For example, a marathon requires longer, slower training than used in the study, and older athletes tend to require longer recovery times. Thus, marathoners and long-distance triathletes may do better with more tapering, as may older athletes.

The following tapering program is based on this study, in which 25 subjects exercised for 60 min at a high intensity level 5 days a week, for 6 weeks, in *one sport*. Thus, this is a good tapering program for single-sport short- or middle-distance events, such as 5-km and 10-km road races.

Naturally, for multisport events, or races that are longer, the tapering schedule should be modified and lengthened. In this case, use the program as a general template to gauge how much you should decrease your exercise over a longer tapering period. The following grids present long and short tapering programs. In the next section, we'll look at a more complete tapering program, a 14-day countdown to a long-distance event.

The 6-Day Taper

Day 1	40 min exercise
Day 2	Complete rest
Day 3	40 min exercise
Day 4	20 min exercise
Day 5	20 min exercise
Day 6	Complete rest
Day 7	Race day

The 3-Day Taper

Day 1	40 min exercise
Day 2	20 min exercise
Day 3	Complete rest
Day 4	Race day

THE 14-DAY COUNTDOWN

Even if your training hasn't been perfect, or you've overtrained a little, the 14 days before a race or organized competition are crucial. It's the critical zone, a period during which it's absolutely essential that you pay attention to some vital areas of your life.

It's an ideal time to tune up your body and your mind, to round out your marathon training to integrate and combine some of the important variables we've talked about in previous chapters, such as mental training, rest, and nutrition.

In the 1989 bestseller *The Seven Habits of Highly Effective People*, Stephen R. Covey calls this process "sharpening the saw." Finishing a long-distance event with physical training only is like trying to chop down a tree with a dull blade. If you take the time in the next 14 days to "sharpen the saw" by giving your body some much-needed rest, doing some mental training, making good nutritional choices, and paying attention to some details, you'll chop down that tree in no time.

Although this countdown is based on tapering for endurance events such as triathlons, marathons, or long-distance cycling, the principles can be applied to any extended competitive event. Whatever your sport, use it as a template for peak performance.

SUNDAY: 14 DAYS TO GO

Training: You should do your last long workout, but not your longest. Train at distances roughly equivalent to half of your longest workout. Some professionals will do their hardest workout on this day, but elite athletes have ideal muscle composition for endurance (predominantly slow-twitch fibers) that allow for quick recovery. The majority of amateurs require more time, so your longest workout should be 3 to 4 weeks before race day. If you feel good, put in a few short surges of speed, just to build confidence.

Mental Training: Besides visualizing while you train, begin to set aside 15 to 30 min every day to spend in a quiet place where you won't be interrupted. Close your eyes and relax. Take deep, slow breaths, inhaling through your mouth and exhaling through your nose. Visualize the starting line. See yourself on the day of the race, relaxed and confident.

You're calm and cool within the hustle and bustle of the crowd. See as much detail as possible, and feel an eager anticipation to meet the challenge that awaits you. If you're not used to meditating, this may seem difficult at first. Persist, as you've done with your physical training, and subsequent sessions will go better.

Nutrition: This is a good time to experiment with your ideal prerace meal. Try eating a high-carbohydrate snack such as a bagel and a banana 60 to 90 min before your long workout to ensure that you don't experience nausea. After your workout, eat a high-carbohydrate, low-fat meal.

Details: If you're doing an out-of-town event, take any essential equipment to a specialty shop for a full safety check. (If you're a triathlete or cyclist, now's a good time for a bicycle tune-up.) You want to give your shop plenty of time in case any major service is needed or parts have to be ordered.

MONDAY: 13 DAYS TO GO

Training: Take the day off and do any shopping you might need to do. If you intend to get new shoes or equipment, do it today so you have ample time to break them in.

Mental Training: Visualize the start of the race. You're at the beach or on the starting line, and the gun goes off. It's rough at first and everyone's crowding you, but once you get some breathing space, you settle into your desired pace.

Nutrition: If you intend to carboload (see chapter 7), you've been following the recommended 70% carbohydrate diet for endurance athletes, and your pantry should be well-stocked with pasta, grains, fruits, and vegetables. If not, do some shopping.

TUESDAY: 12 DAYS TO GO

Training: Do a light cross-training workout today. If cross-training hasn't been part of your regimen, do a 30- to 40-min cardiovascular activity.

Mental Training: By now you should be looking forward to your visualization sessions. They are a peaceful time to anticipate the challenge of the competition in your mind's eye. See yourself at some early point in the race, perhaps waving to spectators along the course. You're feeling great, and your body feels fresh.

Nutrition: If you haven't been taking supplements during your training, consider making a trip to the health food store for a multivitamin supplement with moderate amounts of vitamins C and E, zinc, and beta carotene.

WEDNESDAY: 11 DAYS TO GO

Training: If you've been doing intervals or track training, this should be your last speed workout. Make it short. Do 3- to 5-min intervals 10 to 30 s faster than your planned race pace, with 30-s to 20-min recoveries. If you haven't been doing speed work, perform a short aerobic activity at a steady pace.

Mental Training: Imagine yourself nearing the middle portion of your event. If you plan to compete against your rival, think of the drama starting to unfold.

Nutrition: Are you staying away from high-fat foods like cheese, whole milk, and butter? Make an effort to fine-tune your diet.

Details (equipment): Make a list of all the items you'll need to bring with you to the race, especially if you are traveling out of town. If it is a multisport event, make an equipment checklist for each sport. Don't forget small items like Vaseline® to rub around your armpits for a run, or to dab along your ankles to get your wetsuit off quickly. And don't forget any of the mandatory safety equipment, such as your helmet (or pads, if you're participating in an in-line skating event).

THURSDAY: 10 DAYS TO GO

Training: Train at a comfortable pace for 30 min. If you find these "easy" sessions boring, try a new route or work out with a group or club in your area.

Mental Training: You're just about one-third done in your mind's eye. You're feeling refreshed, taking pride in knowing you've finally made it this far in such great shape.

Nutrition: If you're having trouble digesting a high-carbohydrate diet and are experiencing gas spells, which is a common occurrence, try spacing out your meals during the day.

Details: If you've gotten your equipment, try it out on the road to make sure everything's in working order.

FRIDAY: 9 DAYS TO GO

Training: Work out for 30 min at a comfortable pace.

Mental Training: The halfway mark of any long-distance event is a critical juncture. By then, you should know whether you have the "stuff" or not. Picture yourself halfway into the race feeling vibrant, full of energy, and ready to take on the second half of the course. Sure, you ache a little here and there, but overall, you're in good shape.

Nutrition: Are you keeping well-hydrated? Make sure you drink six to eight 8-oz servings of water a day. If you'll be using a sports drink, energy bar, or carbohydrate gel during your competition, make sure you're well-stocked for the event.

SATURDAY: 8 DAYS TO GO

Training: Take the day off. Go get a tan. If training has taken a toll on your loved ones, use this time to make it up to them.

Mental Training: You're more than halfway done, and the strain of the effort is starting to show. But you see yourself cool and calm under the stress. Shift your focus to your form and the consistent pace you've been keeping.

Nutrition: If you eat out, try a vegetarian restaurant with plenty of healthy, high-carbohydrate dishes, or dine at a restaurant with a "heart-healthy" menu endorsed by the American Heart Association. These dishes are usually low in fat and high in carbs.

SUNDAY: 7 DAYS TO GO

Training: Some endurance athletes prefer to compete in a short-distance event, such as a 10-km race or a sprint-distance triathlon, the week before a long-distance event. If this is your first time competing, I don't recommend it, but if you're a veteran, it's a good way to recharge your training and shake the dust off your legs.

Mental Training: You see yourself at this point in your "mental" race as feeling somewhat tight, but reasonably fresh and energetic. You know that "the wall" is up ahead, but you visualize yourself as strong and confident.

Nutrition: Review your diet for the past week. Have you maintained a diet of at least 70% carbohydrate and cut down on your fat? If you're not getting enough protein, integrate some legumes, egg whites, and low-fat dairy products into your diet. If you haven't been eating right, make a commitment to get your nutritional act together in the coming critical week. You've come too far to let diet stop you from being your very best.

Details (travel): Do you need to make any special travel arrangements to get to the starting line on time? Make sure your travel schedule allows enough time so that you're ready when the gun sounds.

MONDAY: 6 DAYS TO GO

Training: Take the day off. If you feel like you're taking too many days off, or that you're losing the fitness edge you've worked so hard for, remember your body needs time to fully recover from all the damage to muscle fibers you've done over the last few months. Relax and concentrate on your mental training.

Mental Training: Visualize yourself two-thirds into your event. See yourself feeling reenergized as it dawns on you that you have only one-third left to go.

Nutrition: You may want to consider shopping for a high-carbohydrate loading/recovery drink that makes it easy to ingest large amounts of carbs without all the bulk.

Details: If you've traveled to an event and have gotten there a few days early, check out the race course or track. Don't bother with a detailed topographic analysis or worry about every little pothole. Just get a feel for the course and the kind of conditions you'll be dealing with. Also, go to a local supermarket and buy any food and supplies you need for the coming week.

TUESDAY: 5 DAYS TO GO

Training: Do a light cross-training workout, preferably swimming or some other nonimpact exercise.

Mental Training: If this is your first long event, you won't know what it feels like to hit the wall or "bonk" until it happens. If you've done the race before, you know that you have to be mentally tough to break through it. Imagine yourself having that toughness, that look of determination etched in your face as you bear down.

Nutrition: Don't panic if you notice you've gained a few pounds. The extra carbohydrates and water are what you need to get you through the event.

Details (massage): Schedule a massage session sometime within the next day. It'll help you get the kinks out and stay relaxed. Let your massage therapist know what you're doing Sunday so that he or she takes it easy on you. You don't want a massage that will cause soreness—just soothing, relaxing therapy.

WEDNESDAY: 4 DAYS TO GO

Training: Perform some easy, nonimpact physical activity such as swimming or beach tanning. (The latter is my choice in Kona before the Ironman.)

Mental Training: If music inspires you, try listening to your favorite inspirational song and visualize yourself nearing the last few miles of your race. You've conquered the wall, and the spring is back in your body. While others are wilting from the effort, you're passing up people like an Indy race car.

Nutrition: If you didn't step up your carbohydrate intake earlier in the week, now is the time to load up on carbs to increase your muscle glycogen to full capacity. The more full the fuel tank on race day, the better off you'll be.

THURSDAY: 3 DAYS TO GO

Training: Perform an easy cardiovascular workout for 15 min. Concentrate on your form and on staying loose. You may feel the urge for a last-minute hard workout, but it won't do you any good at this point, and it might do harm.

Mental Training: Whatever your event, see yourself nearing the end of your race. In your mind, you see yourself as tight and tired, but you've got your second wind now, and you're practically home.

Nutrition: Continue carbo loading, but don't get all your carbohydrates from sports beverages. Although they are excellent supplements, you also need the nutritious complex carbohydrates in vegetables, fruits, and grains.

FRIDAY: 2 DAYS TO GO

Training: Take the day off.

Mental Training: What a feeling to be able to see the spectators lining the street and the distant finish line!

Nutrition: Again, if you're finding all those carbohydrates difficult to digest, the key is frequent snacking during the day. What you eat today is more important than what you eat tomorrow, so don't deviate from your tried-and-true high-carbohydrate favorites.

Details (sleep): Try to get to bed early tonight to prepare you for the hectic weekend. After making any last-minute race arrangements, settle down for a quiet, relaxing evening.

SATURDAY: 1 DAY TO GO

Training: If you work out at all, don't do it for more than 10 min. A very short cardiovascular workout might loosen you up if you feel tense.

Mental Training: Visualize the finish line within sight. The crowds are cheering you on, and you cross the line, setting a new personal best for yourself. Imagine what it feels like. Concentrate and focus on the positive emotions you'll feel.

Nutrition: Eat dinner early so you can get a good night's sleep. As long as you stick to plenty of carbohydrates and fluids, what you eat tonight shouldn't affect your performance adversely.

Details (equipment): Pick out your race day outfit and pack your gym bag with your equipment. Lay out all your clothes, check your equipment (especially your bicycle, if applicable), and make sure you have everything you need. Prepare and freeze water bottles or sports drinks.

SUNDAY: RACE DAY

Nutrition: Wake up at least 2 hr before the event, and eat a small high-carbohydrate meal 60 to 90 min before the race. Drink water or a sports drink, too.

Mental Preparation: Chances are you'll be pretty hyper on race morning. This can cause digestive problems, as well as turn you into a bundle of nerves in the few hours prior to the start. Try to relax. Listen to soothing music, something classical or New Age. Think of all the heroic reasons you're competing at this event, and feel grateful for the opportunity you have today to bring your purpose to fruition. If you're so inclined, say a prayer.

Details (starting line): Keep your sweats on for as long as possible. Expect the starting area to be crowded, so give yourself enough time to get a crack at the porta-potty.

The Race: Keep a steady pace, stay focused, and drink plenty of fluids. When it gets tough, think about all you've done in the last 2 weeks to "sharpen the saw." All the training, the nutritious diet, and the mental preparation will help you get back that edge to perform at your peak.

DEALING WITH A COMMON RACE ANNOYANCE

You see it all the time at a triathlon or road race, usually in the first few miles of the run: athletes slowing to a crawl, grabbing their sides, and grimacing in pain. There is nothing quite as upsetting as having to slow to a crawl on the first mile of a road race simply because your side feels like you're about to give birth to an alien, à la Sigourney Weaver.

Sidestitches are a common difficulty during competition, and no one seems to know exactly what causes them. Some experts feel they may be caused by drinking too many fluids or going out too fast. I've managed to avoid them by watching my fluid intake and pacing myself at the beginning of a run. Here are a few simple precautions you can take to avoid sidestitches.

- Don't take in excessive amounts of food or fluids prior to hard running, and avoid fatty foods. Everyone digests at a different rate, but time your meals so that you don't feel like a water balloon with legs.
- Stay loose and relaxed. If you're nervous at the start of that PR-busting run, the added tension could hamper your breathing or cause you to go out too fast.
- Some experts say sidestitches may be caused by weaknesses in the abdominals. The abdominal exercises illustrated in chapter 4 will help reinforce this area of your body.
- Don't race or train beyond your fitness level. Unrealistic speeds may bring on sidestitches.

If you get a sidestitch, here are a few ways to cope.

- Slow down or walk it off. You may be pushing yourself too hard.
- Breathe deeply. Concentrate on forceful exhalations. Try changing your breathing pattern. Grunting, coughing, or other obnoxious noises may help.
- Massage the area that hurts. If your internal organs are not getting enough blood, or if your diaphragm is being irritated, this may help relieve the tension.
- Although it may be the last thing you want to do in a race, stop, lie down, and put your feet up in the air. Sidestitches sometimes mimic the symptoms of a heart attack, so if the pain doesn't go away, seek medical attention immediately.

ERIN'S DAY

My biggest disappointment in a race came, not so much as a result of my lack of fitness, but as a result of an incredible running performance—unmatched to this day—by Erin Baker during the 1990 Canadian Ironman. I remember my thoughts as I approached the marathon turnaround point. *There's no way she can catch me* now. *This one's in the bag.* I was feeling good, and I had that spring in my legs that told me I was knocking off the miles at a good pace. I knew that I was at least 10 min ahead of her at the beginning of the run, a lead that—barring a catastrophe—I was sure I'd keep. I'd had a good swim and an excellent bike, and Erin was miles behind me. Or so I thought.

Feeling as though I had been jolted back to reality after daydreaming my way across a busy intersection, I made the turnaround, only to see Erin Baker just a few yards away.

It was a sobering, shocking, demoralizing, devastating experience. As Erin gained ground on me at a remarkable pace, all I could do was watch and swallow my pride. I was going as fast as I could, yet I looked like I was standing still. In the few moments it took for her to take the lead, and my victory, away from me, I wished her well: "Wow, you're having a great run," I said. My words of support belied my true feelings. I felt like crying.

POSTEVENT ANALYSIS

Almost everyone has had the experience of falling short of expectations, whether it be in a schoolroom or in the athletic arena. Perhaps you failed to set a new PR because you overestimated your fitness level. Maybe—like Erin on that day in 1990—your rival was being interviewed by the press by the time you finished. Whatever the nature of your disappointment, chances are it will be emotionally and mentally tough to deal with.

This emotional turmoil is an unfortunate consequence of competition. Because of all the months you spent training and preparing for competition, it's only natural that a subpar performance will be frustrating.

How we come away from a competition has dramatic effects on our subsequent performances. Instead of letting that race in Canada ruin my career, I stepped back to do some postevent analysis in the days following the event. I made a conscious attempt to gain some objectivity, and I realized that my performance was good and Erin's was spectacular. (She had a faster run than *any man* that day, including her husband, pro triathlete Scott Molina.)

REBOUND FOR SUCCESS

Serious athletes tend to have a particularly tough time coping with disappointing performances and doing a truly objective postevent analysis. West Coast psychologist Kathleen Zechmeister, PhD, works with athletes in the San Diego area to help them rebound from competitive setbacks. In her practice, she uses a method known as cognitive reconstructing to help athletes see the difference between how you look at the failure and the facts. This is done in five steps that use writing as a tool for self-examination.

"Thoughts and emotions occur simultaneously," says Dr. Zechmeister. "For example, right after a poor performance, there's always a lot of reaction. Usually it is clouded with emotions that are self-critical and negative. Cognitive reconstructing helps you separate the negative emotions and judgments from what actually happened."

Dr. Zechmeister suggests you try this postevent exercise immediately after a competition in which you feel you have done poorly. Your writing should be free-form, with no word or time limitations.

Step 1

Draw a line down the middle of a sheet of paper. On the left-hand side, write a factual account of the event in which you performed poorly. The account should include such things as splits, weather conditions, mechanical problems, race course conditions, heart rate, or any other available data that you can recall or produce.

Step 2

On the right-hand side, write your reactions to the facts. How did you feel during each portion of the event? Describe your moods and any self-criticism that may have been going through your head.

Step 3

Compare the facts on the left side with your judgments and emotions on the right side. Ask yourself: Did you expect to do a lot better? Were those realistic expectations? Although you may not have reached your highest expectations, did you achieve any other objectives? (For example, although you may not have won your age group, where did you place? Was it in the top three? Top ten? Top 25%?)

Step 4

Rewrite your race report to include the positive facts that may have surfaced, leaving out the emotional judgments.

Step 5

Compare your new race report with your feelings during the race (seen in step 2) as well as with the negative feelings you may now have about the event.

Ask yourself: Did I really do that poorly? Was it the disaster that I had originally painted?

"*Usually* after doing this, most athletes feel somewhat positive and less disappointed," says Dr. Zechmeister, "but at least you've stepped away from 'should haves' and 'could haves,' which take away from your positive belief system, and replaced them with the facts. I've found that if competitive athletes don't do this kind of analysis about a disappointing performance, they'll tend to take this kind of mental garbage into the next race."

"I call it the reality versus the mythology of a situation," she says. "It also helps you to see that whatever happened wasn't final, that this was one day out of your race career. The way people improve is by understanding that a bad race was just a moment in time. People tend to be more upset and self-critical about themselves than is warranted. Once you go beyond that, you can look at the factors that led up to that setback and learn from it."

WHAT NOW?

Sometimes it doesn't matter how well you do; you still feel bummed that something you've trained for, something you've put your heart into for so long, is finally over.

There is a common expression used among veteran triathletes to describe the period immediately following the Gatorade® Ironman World Championship Triathlon, traditionally the last big race of the season. We call it the "After-Ironman Depression Syndrome." Because of the long distances involved (2.4-mi swim, 112-mi bike, and 26.2-mi run) and a high level of international competition, professional triathletes put extraordinary effort into preparing for this race.

When it is all over, win or lose, finish or not, there is always a sense of loss. Yet, because it is a part of my lifestyle, I have learned to weather it, to move on and get back to living, to thrive on other new challenges. I treat this time not as something permanent, but as a natural lull that will inevitably pass.

This approach of treating competitions as integrative tools for your life can be applied repeatedly. Lulls will even occur after a particularly satisfying performance. Look upon them as a naturally occurring phenomenon that is a normal part of your life.

THE NEXT STEP

Certainly, after completing a competitive event or achieving a formidable fitness goal, you deserve a rest. Besides the steps you need to take to recover physically, you also need to reenergize yourself on a mental and even on a spiritual level.

The next step you take is, of course, up to you. After you've conquered some new fitness ground, you may choose to have fun and explore new territory and exciting new sports, such as in-line skating or mountain biking. Perhaps you'd like to try something totally different, such as skydiving or snowboarding. Or, you may decide to begin the whole process again and shoot for higher ground in the same sport.

As an active woman or female athlete, the fitness choices are endless, the frontiers ever changing, and the rewards incredibly gratifying.

Whatever form it may take, good luck on your quest for peak fitness.

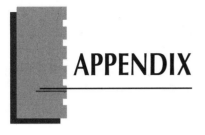

APPENDIX

REFERRAL SERVICES

The following listings can help you if you'd like further information or referrals on these subjects.

Massage

The American Massage
 Therapy Association
820 Davis St., Ste. 100
Evanston, IL 60201
708-864-0123

Rolf Institute
205 Canyon Blvd.
Boulder, CO 80302
800-530-8875

Nutrition

To find a certified nutritionist in your area, call the American Dietetic Association's Referral System between the hours of 9 a.m. and 4 p.m., Central Standard Time:

The American Dietetic Association
216 W. Jackson Blvd.
Chicago, IL 60606-6995
800-366-1655

Pilates

If you are interested in the Pilates Method described in chapter 3 and would like to find a studio in your area, contact:

The Institute of the Pilates Method
1807 2nd St., #28
Sante Fe, NM 87505
505-988-1990

Sports Nutrition

The Gatorade® Company offers free literature on various sports nutrition topics, including an excellent brochure entitled *Nutrition Fundamentals for Performance* and a comprehensive *Swimmer's Diet* booklet. They can also provide you with up-to-date information on current sports nutrition research or point you to other resources.

Gatorade® Sports Science Institute
The Quaker Oats Company
P.O. Box 9005
Chicago, IL 60604-9005
312-222-7704

NATIONAL ORGANIZATIONS

The following are national organizations that specialize in some of the sports discussed throughout the book. A national organization can help you familiarize yourself with other athletes, coaches, and events in your area.

Aerobics

The Aerobics and Fitness
  Association of America
15250 Ventura Blvd., Ste. 200
Sherman Oaks, CA 91403
800-445-5950

American Aerobics Association
  International
P.O. Box 633
Richbora, PA 18954
215-598-0608

International Dance-Exercise
Association
6190 Cornerstone Ct. E., Ste. 204
San Diego, CA 92121-3773
800-999-4332

Cross-Country Skiing

The Cross-Country Ski Areas Association
259 Bolton Rd.
Winchester, NH 03470
603-239-4341

Cycling

United States Cycling
Federation
One Olympic Plaza
Colorado Springs, CO
80909-5775
719-578-4581

League of American Bicyclists
190 W. Ostend St., Ste. 120
Baltimore, MD 21230-3755
410-539-3399

Rails to Trails Conservancy
913 W. Holmes, Ste. 145
Lansing, MI 48910
517-393-6022

ULTRA Marathon Cycling
Association
P.O. Box 53
Canyon, TX 79015
806-499-3290

Women's Cycling Network
P.O. Box 302
Coraopolis, PA 15108
412-262-7265

In-Line Skating

International In-Line Skating Association
P.O. Box 15482
Atlanta, GA 30333
404-728-9707

Mountain Biking

NORBA
One Olympic Plaza
Colorado Springs, CO 80909
719-578-4717

Rowing

The U.S. Rowing Association
201 S. Capital Ave., Ste. 400
Indianapolis, IN 46225
317-237-5656

Running

USA Track & Field
P.O. Box 120
Indianapolis, IN 46206
317-261-0500

American Running & Fitness
  Association
4405 East West Hwy., #405
Bethesda, MD 20814
301-913-9517

Road Runners Club of America
1150 S. Washington St. #250
Alexandria, VA 22314
703-836-0558

Swimming

United States Swimming
1 Olympic Plaza
Colorado Springs, CO 80909
719-578-4578

United States Masters
  Swimming
2 Peter Ave.
Rutland, MA 01543
508-886-6631

Triathlon

Triathlon Federation USA
3595 E. Fountain Blvd.
Colorado Springs, CO
  80910
719-597-9090

Tri-Canada
1154 W. 24th St.
N. Vancouver, BC V7P2J2
604-987-0092

Walking

American Racewalk Association
P.O. Box 1323
Boulder, CO 80308-1323
303-447-0156

OTHER RESOURCES

The following are vendors and organizations that help supply you with equipment or information on race events.

Surgical Tubing

To purchase surgical tubing with handles for strength training, including a brochure that describes and illustrates various exercises, contact:

SPRI
1684 Barclay Blvd.
Buffalo Grove, IL 60089
800-222-7774

Indoor Rowing Competitions

For more information and a listing of indoor rowing competitions in your area, contact:

Concept II Incorporated
RR #1, Box 1100
Morrisville, VT 05661-9727
800-245-5676

Race Information

Race information is routinely published in the periodicals for each sport. For information on the triathlons mentioned in the book, contact:

Ironman Mainland Office
  World Triathlon Corporation
43309 U.S. Hwy. 19N
Tarpon Springs, FL 34689
813-942-4767

Danskin Race Series
111 W. 40th, 18th Floor
New York, NY 10018
800-452-9526

Strength Training Video

To order *Strength Training for Total Body Fitness*, a great video on Diane Buchta's comprehensive strength training program (described in chapter 4) starring Mark Allen and yours truly, send $29.95* plus $4.87 for shipping and handling to:

Strength Training for Total Body Fitness
P.O. Box 15872
Beverly Hills, CA 90209
800-977-FITT

*California residents add $2.25 sales tax.

PERIODICALS

Bicycling
33 E. Minor St.
Emmaus, PA 18098
800-441-7761

Competitor and *Competitor for Women*
214 S. Cedros Ave.
Solana Beach, CA 92075
619-793-2711

InLine
P.O. Box 527
Mt. Morris, IL 61054
800-877-5281

Inside Triathlon
1830 N. 55th St.
Boulder, CO 80301
800-825-8793

Peak Running Performance
P.O. Box 128036
Nashville, TN 37212
615-383-1071

Runner's World
33 E. Minor St.
Emmaus, PA 18098
800-441-7761

Running Times
98 N. Washington St.
Boston, MA 02114
617-367-2228

Skiing
P.O. Box 54180
Boulder, CO 80322
800-825-5552

Swim Magazine
228 Nevada St.
El Segundo, CA 90245
310-607-9956

Triathlete
121 Second St.
San Francisco, CA 94105
800-441-1666

Velo-News
1830 N. 55th St.
Boulder, CO 80301
800-825-8793

Walking
9-11 Harcourt St.
Boston, MA 02116-6439
800-678-0881

Winning, Bicycling Racing Illustrated
121 Second St.
San Francisco, CA 94105
800-441-1666

Women's Sports and Fitness Magazine
P.O. Box 472
Mt. Morris, IL 61054
800-877-5281

BOOKS

The Heart Rate Monitor Book, Sally Edwards, Polar, 1992.

Lore of Running, Tim Noakes, Leisure Press, 1991.

Nancy Clark's Sports Nutrition Guidebook, Nancy Clark, Leisure Press, 1990.

Nutrition for Women, the Complete Guide, Elizabeth Somer, Henry Holt & Co., 1993.

Serious Training for Serious Athletes, Rob Sleamaker, Human Kinetics, 1989.

Swim, Bike, Run, Glenn Town & Todd Kearney, Human Kinetics, 1994.

Triathlon for Women, Sally Edwards, *Triathlete* Magazine, 1992.

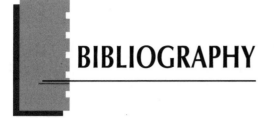

BIBLIOGRAPHY

American College of Sports Medicine. (1993). *The recommended quantity and quality of exercise for developing and maintaining cardiorespiratory and muscular fitness in healthy adults.* Indianapolis: Author.

Arthritis Foundation, Arthritis Today. (1994). *Arthritis today research supplement* (p. 15). Atlanta: Author.

Boyden, T.W. (1993). Effects of resistance training on cholesterol levels of females. *Archives of Internal Medicine,* **153**, 16-21.

Brooks, D., & Copeland-Brooks, C. (Jan. 11, 1993). Uncovering the myths of abdominal exercises. *Idea Today,* p. 42.

Covey, S.R. (1989). *The seven habits of highly effective people.* New York: Simon & Schuster.

Coyle, E. (1988). Carbohydrates and athletic performance. *Sports Science Exchange,* **1**(7).

Davis, J.M., Lamb, D.R., Burgess, W.A., & Bartoli, W.P. (1987). Accumulation of deuterium oxide in body fluids after ingestion of d20-labeled beverages. *Journal of Applied Physiology,* **23**, 2060-2066.

Friel, J. (1993, December). Pumping iron for pr's. *MastersSports,* 1.

Gavenas, M.L. (1993, March). The beauty of strength. *Weight Watchers Magazine,* 16.

Gisolfi, C.J. (1990). Human intestinal water absorption: Direct versus indirect measurements. *American Journal of Physiology,* **54**, 216-222.

Hay, Louise (1987). *You can heal your life.* Santa Monica, CA: Hay House.

Heaney, R.P. (1987). The role of calcium in prevention and treatment of osteoporosis. *The Physician and Sportsmedicine,* **20**, 83-88.

Hubbarb, R.W., Sandick, B.L., Mathew, W.T., Francesconi, R.P., Sampson, J.B., Dorkot, M.J., Maller, O., & Engell, D.B. (1984). Voluntary dehydration and water. *Journal of Applied Physiology,* **21**, 868-875.

Institute of Nutrition and Fitness. (1993, May). Choosing the right exercise. *Good Housekeeping,* 134.

Ivy, J.L., Katz, A.L., Cutler, C.L., Sherman, W.M., & Coyle, E.F. (1988). Muscle glycogen syntheses after exercise: Effect of time of carbohydrate ingestion. *Journal of Applied Physiology,* **88,** 1480.

Kaufmann, E. (1993, June). The new case for woman power. *Good Health,* 19.

Mangi, R., Jokl, P., & Dayton, O.W. (1979). *The runner's complete medical guide.* New York: Summit Books.

Mann, M. (1992). Static active stretching training for a healthy back. *The Spine Surgeon,* **12,** 18.

Mora, J.M. (1993, April). Tapering tips. *Running Times,* 19.

Nardo, D. (1992). *The encyclopedia of health: Exercise.* New York: Chelsea House.

Ryan, M. (1992, November). Muscles and the right nutrients for resistance training. *VeloNews,* 90.

Sherman, W.M. (1989). Effects of 4 h preexercise carbohydrate feedings on cycling performance. *Medicine and Science in Sports and Exercise,* **21,** 598.

Sherman, W.M. (1989). Pre-event nutrition. *Sports Science Exchange,* **1**(12).

Sherman, W.M. (1991). Carbohydrate feedings 1 h before exercise improves cycling performances. *American Journal of Clinical Nutrition,* **54,** 866-870.

Sleamaker, R. (1989). *Serious training for serious athletes.* Champaign, IL: Leisure Press.

Sudi, M. (1991). *Personal trainer manual, the resource for fitness instructors.* San Diego: American Council on Exercise and Rebok University Press.

Sullivan, M.E. (1993, January). Stretch—it feels good. *Current Health,* 4.

Town, G. (1985). *The science of triathlon training and competition.* Champaign, IL: Human Kinetics.

Work, J.A. (1991, January). Are java junkies poor sports? *The Physician and Sportsmedicine,* 83-88.

Zawadzki, K.M., Yaspelskis, B.B. III, and Ivy, J.L. (1992). Carbohydrate-protein complex increases the rate of muscle glycogen storage after exercise. *Journal of Applied Physiology,* **92,** 1854.

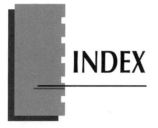

INDEX

Note: Page numbers in italics refer to figures or tables.

ABOUT THE AUTHORS

Paula Newby-Fraser may be the most highly fit and finely tuned athlete ever. This eight-time Gatorade® Ironman Triathlon world champion is also the Ironman world record holder with a time of 8:55:24. In fact, she owns seven of the ten best-ever women's Ironman times. Few, if any, athletes dominate a sport as Paula has for the last decade.

Yet it wasn't always so. Paula confesses to being an "out-of-shape couch potato" until age 20. But once she embraced the concept of peak fitness, she left South Africa and moved to the United States to pursue her dream of becoming a professional triathlete. She won her first Ironman World Championship in 1986, and since that time she has continued to surpass her competition in triathlons and other distance races around the world.

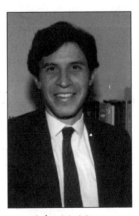

Paula Newby-Fraser

In 1990 The Women's Sports Foundation honored Paula with the Professional Sportswoman of the Year Award, and *Triathlete Magazine* voted her Triathlete of the Year. She was named Professional Female Athlete of the Decade by the *Los Angeles Times*, and *ABC's Wide World of Sports* proclaimed her the Greatest All-Around Female Athlete in the World in 1989.

John M. Mora

Paula understands how difficult it can be to adhere to a training program, so she coauthored this book to help other women who want to rise above their current fitness levels and realize their athletic potential.

Paula lives and trains in Encinitas, a town on the California coastline.

John M. Mora is a nationally known sports, health and fitness, and medical writer. He has published more than 100 articles in magazines such as *American Health, Women's Sports and Fitness,* and *Runner's World.* He is president of John M. Mora Creative Communications, a company that specializes in writing promotional copy for businesses in the health and fitness industry.

John has competed across the country in 8 marathons, 50 running and cycling events, and 30 triathlons. He lives in LaGrange Highlands, Illinois, a suburb of Chicago.

MORE BOOKS FOR MULTISPORT ATHLETES

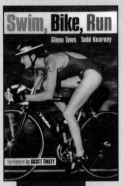

Glenn Town and Todd Kearney
Foreword by Scott Tinley

1994 • Paper • 240 pp • Item PTOW0513
ISBN 0-87322-513-9 • $16.95 ($24.95 Canadian)

**SERIOUS Training for
Endurance Athletes**
(Second Edition)
Rob Sleamaker and Ray Browning

1996 • Paper • 320 pp
Item PSLE0644 • ISBN 0-87322-644-5
$15.95 ($23.95 Canadian)

**Time-Saving Training for
Multisport Athletes**
Rick Niles
Foreword by Karen Smyers

1997 • Paper • 192 pp
Item PNIL0538 • ISBN 0-88011-538-6
$16.95 ($24.95 Canadian)

Marc Evans
Foreword by Scott Tinley

1997 • Paper • 240 pp • Item PEVA0938
ISBN 0-87322-938-X • $19.95 ($29.95 Canadian)

30-day money-back guarantee!

Prices subject to change.

Human Kinetics
*The Premier Publisher for
Sports & Fitness*
http://www.humankinetics.com/

2335

To request more information or to place your order,
U.S. customers call **TOLL FREE 1-800-747-4457**.
Customers outside the U.S. place your order using the
appropriate telephone number/address
shown in the front of this book.

RESOURCES FOR FITNESS ENTHUSIASTS AND COMPETITORS

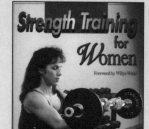

James A. Peterson, Cedric X. Bryant, and Susan L. Peterson
Foreword by Willye White
1996 • Paper • 168pp • Item PPET0752
ISBN 0-87322-522-2 • $15.95 ($22.95 Canadian)

Cross-Training for Sports
Gary T. Moran and
George H. McGlynn
1997 • Paper • 240 pp
Item PMOR0493 • ISBN 0-88011-493-2
$19.95 ($29.95 Canadian)

Sport Stretch
(Second Edition)
Michael J. Alter
1997 • Paper • 232 pp
Item PALT0823 • ISBN 0-88011-823-7
$15.95 ($23.95 Canadian)

Nancy Clark's Sports Nutrition Guidebook
(Second Edition)
Nancy Clark
1997 • Paper • 464 pp
Item PCLA0730 • ISBN 0-87322-730-1
$15.95 ($22.95 Canadian)

John Yacenda
1995 • Paper • 168 pp • Item PYAC0770
ISBN 0-87322-770-0 • $14.95 ($19.95 Canadian)

30-day money-back guarantee!

Prices subject to change.

Human Kinetics
The Premier Publisher for
Sports & Fitness
http://www.humankinetics.com/

2335

To request more information or to place your order,
U.S. customers call **TOLL FREE 1-800-747-4457**.
Customers outside the U.S. place your order using the
appropriate telephone number/address
shown in the front of this book.